Dementia Care

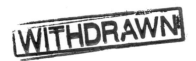

Dementia Care

A Practical Photographic Guide

James Grealy   PhD, RN, Grad. Dip. Psych-Mental Health

Helen McMullen   BSc (Occupational Therapy)

Julia Grealy   RN, BA Hons, MBA

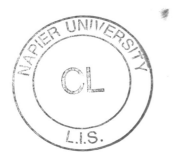
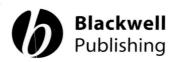

Blackwell
Publishing

© 2005 by Blackwell Publishing Ltd

Editorial offices:
Blackwell Publishing Ltd, 9600 Garsington Road, Oxford OX4 2DQ, UK
  Tel: +44 (0)1865 776868
Blackwell Publishing Inc., 350 Main Street, Malden, MA 02148-5020, USA
  Tel: +1 781 388 8250
Blackwell Publishing Asia Pty Ltd, 550 Swanston Street, Carlton, Victoria 3053, Australia
  Tel: +61 (0)3 8359 1011

The right of the Author to be identified as the Author of this Work has been asserted in accordance
with the Copyright, Designs and Patents Act 1988.

First published 2004 under the title *Everyday Dementia Care: A Practical Photographic Guide Including
Environmental Management* (ISBN: 0-9756-8441-8), by Big Kidz Pty Ltd, Australia
First published 2005 under the title *Dementia Care*, by Blackwell Publishing Ltd

ISBN-13: 978-14051-3428-6
ISBN-10: 1-4051-3428-3

Library of Congress Cataloging-in-Publication Data

Grealy, James.
    Dementia care: a practical photographic guide/James Grealy, Helen McMullen, Julia Grealy.
       p.   ; cm.
    Includes bibliographical references and index.
    ISBN-13: 978-1-4051-3428-6 (alk. paper)
    ISBN-10: 1-4051-3428-3 (alk. paper)
   1. Dementia – Patients – Care.   2. Dementia – Nursing.   3. Dementia – Patients – Care – Pictorial works.
4. Dementia – Nursing – Pictorial works.
    [DNLM: 1. Dementia – Aged – Pictorial Works.   2. Long – term Care – methods – Aged – Pictorial Works.
WT 17 G786d 2006]   I. McMullen, Helen.   II. Grealy, Julia.   III. Title.

RC521.G74   2006
616.8′3–dc22   2005008558

A catalogue record for this title is available from the British Library

Set in 11/13pt Helvetica
by Graphicraft Limited, Hong Kong
Printed and bound in India
by Replika Press Pvt, Ltd, Kundli

The publisher's policy is to use permanent paper from mills that operate a sustainable forestry policy,
and which has been manufactured from pulp processed using acid-free and elementary chlorine-free
practices. Furthermore, the publisher ensures that the text paper and cover board used have met acceptable
environmental accreditation standards.

For further information on Blackwell Publishing, visit our website:
www.blackwellnursing.com

Contents

4   The Interaction   97

Disclaimer

This resource has been prepared by the authors and C&G Education and Research Pty Ltd as part of the tasks undertaken for the project entitled 'Resistance to Care', funded by the WorkCover Corporation Grants Scheme. Whilst all due care has been taken in collecting, collating and interpreting information relevant to the care for older people, some omissions may have occurred. The statements and opinions contained in this resource are given in good faith and in the belief that they are not false or misleading.

Although this resource has been partially or fully funded by the WorkCover Grants Scheme, it does not necessarily represent the views of WorkCover Corporation. The authors, C&G Education and Research Pty Ltd, and WorkCover Corporation do not undertake responsibility in any way whatsoever to any person or organisation in respect of the resource, including any errors or omissions therein, arising through negligence or otherwise, however caused.

This resource is not the only Occupational Health, Safety and Welfare resource available for those who care for older people, but has been tailored to include and consider situational factors that are particularly relevant to this industry/group.

Foreword

Criticisms of residential care recur frequently, usually with lurid newspaper headlines of mistreatment or neglect. But there is another side to this. The media neglect to tell the public the facts about the many dedicated staff who work long hours to provide quality care. Rewards are small but meaningful – a resident's smile, improvement in daily functioning, gratitude from the family, better quality of life.

Of course, there are residential settings where care is less than acceptable. The difference in the quality of care of persons in the later stages of dementia lies principally in the staff – their attitudes, their personal attributes, their knowledge and their skill. Common sense, a strong back and a big heart are important, as are patience, compassion and humanity. But these are not enough.

Care staff need knowledge about the conditions that affect the residents for whom they are caring, about how best to communicate with those whose abilities to understand are diminished, about the appropriate techniques to handle people with dementia who are resistive to care. Technique can make all the difference between a pleasant exchange that is rewarding to the care staff member and to the person with dementia, and an interaction marred by mutual antagonism, resistance to care and, in extreme cases, aggression.

This book on dementia care is a practical, hands on, easy to read guide for the professional or family carer on looking after a person in the later stages of dementia. For example, how do you encourage a nursing home resident to release the rail that she is grasping tightly, without using force to unclench her fingers? How do you make the environment friendly and conducive to pleasurable interaction? How do you assist residents to eat from their own plate, using cutlery in a manner which they would find dignified? What strategies make for good communication between a care staff member and a person in the later stages of dementia? Answers to these questions and many others are included in this book.

The book has an easy to follow layout, generous illustrations and clear explanations. Practitioners who provide hands-on care for people in the late stages of dementia can learn and benefit from reading this. Recommended.

Henry Brodaty
Professor of Psychogeriatrics
University of New South Wales
Chairman
Alzheimer's Disease International

Acknowledgements and Expert Review

This book was produced as part of the 2003–2004 WorkCover Corporation South Australia grant-funded project: Prevention and Management of Resistance to Care in Dementia Care.

This project was conducted under the auspice of an industry committee comprising Aged and Community Services (South Australia) and the Aged Care Association of Australia (South Australia). The Resistance to Care Steering Committee was a sub-committee of the Occupational Health and Safety Committee of the Association of Community Services Inc. and the Aged Care Association of Australia (SA) Inc. Committee members included:

- Peta Saundry, ElderCare Inc.
- Judith Sheidow, Churches of Christ
- Lynn Richardson, ACH Group
- Lyn Bertram, ACH Group
- Lyn Kendricks, ACH Group
- Donna Cox, Alwyndor Aged Care Centre
- Jim Kleszyk, Helping Hand Aged Care Inc.
- Christine Racar, Masonic Homes Inc.
- Betty Hurrell, Wesley Uniting Inc.
- Anna Weise, North Eastern Community Nursing Home
- Angela Sparrow, WorkCover Corporation
- Sue Hutton, Port Adelaide Central Mission

Ethics approval

Ethics approval for the research and implementation project was granted by the ElderCare Inc. Ethics Committee, ElderCare Inc., Wayville, South Australia.

Expert review

Expert review was provided by the Gerontic Nursing Clinical School, ACEBAC La Trobe University Victoria:

- Professor Rhonda Nay, Director of Gerontic Nursing Clinical School and ACEBAC
- Dr Susan Koch, Coordinator of Studies, Gerontic Nursing Clinical School, Co-director ACEBAC

Other expert review

Individuals providing expert review of this book included:

- Sandra (Sam) Davis, PhD (The Environment)
- Revd Jim Spiker, Coordinating Chaplain, ElderCare Inc. (The Care Staff)
- Resistance to Care Steering Committee
- Linda Nazarko, Nurse Consultant, Richmond and Twickenham Primary Care Trust

Gratitude

Our sincere gratitude is expressed to everyone involved in this state-wide project.

Particular thanks must be expressed to the participating twelve residential care facilities for older people:

- The residents and their guardians
- The staff
- The management
- The site champions

Project management:

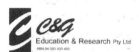

Funded by:

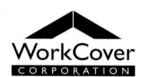

Auspice of:

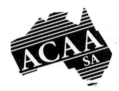

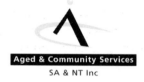

Purpose of Book

The care staff member and person with dementia have a reciprocal relationship and, as such, the care staff member's exposure to Resistance to Care (RTC) is significantly related to the unmet needs of the person with dementia. By identifying the unmet needs of the person with dementia and then acting to either directly meet these needs or facilitating a meeting of these needs can help diminish RTC behaviours. This book has been designed to be applicable across all aspects of dementia care settings, including acute, sub-acute, nursing home, care home and community. The book also seeks to encourage care staff to view the older person with dementia as an individual who has their own individual needs. Consequently, the older person with dementia in this book is referred to by her name, Molly, rather than a patient, resident, client or family member, and the care staff member is referred to by their name. It must be remembered that all persons involved in the care of the person with dementia are care staff members, whether a medical officer, nurse, personal care worker, or pastoral care worker.

The book uses photographs to illustrate some of the main aspects of the ageing process, such as range of movement and reflexes, specific care techniques designed to prevent or manage RTC and also some photographs of common resistive behaviours.

This book has four aims:

(1) To provide an introduction to dementia care.
   This book provides a unique view of dementia care by using a risk management approach. The book has been written with an equal focus on the care staff member and the person with dementia. This is not about competing rights but about getting it right for everyone.

(2) To provide a base level of education for new care staff members in dementia.
   This book has been written in plain English to promote a common understanding. Consequently, in some parts of the book precise scientific terms have been replaced with common language. This book has been designed for care staff of people with dementia and so it includes a self-directed education package located at the end of the book. This education package takes the care staff member through each section. On completion of the education package the care staff member will have a good understanding of person-centred dementia care approaches, risks involved in care and how to prevent and manage these risks involved in care.

(3) To assist in identifying the triggers that elicit RTC.
   The book is designed to immerse you in the world of the person with dementia. This world is based on four variables:
   (i) The person
   (ii) The care staff member

(iii) The interaction
(iv) The environment
As the care staff member you often have the opportunity to influence these variables in a way that increases or decreases the meaning of the world to the person with dementia. By understanding this world, these four variables, and how you influence them can help you start to meet the unmet needs of the person with dementia.

(4) To provide strategies to prevent and/or reduce RTC, or when RTC does occur, provide strategies to manage the behaviours.

This book originated from a project designed to reduce care staff injury in dementia care. Consequently, this book includes a tool designed to describe the behaviours of unmet needs of the person with dementia that occur during care and rates these behaviours in terms of the risk of injury to the care staff member. There is no universal agreement regarding the language used to describe behaviours in dementia care. This book discusses behavioural descriptors and provides the care staff member with four groups of descriptors used in discussing RTC.

Meet the Characters

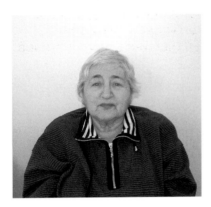

Molly is an 80-year-old person with Alzheimer's type dementia.
Molly is in the early part of stage 2 of dementia.

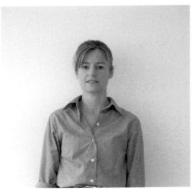

Angela is a 40-year-old care staff member.
Angela sometimes poses in some photographs to demonstrate some care techniques.

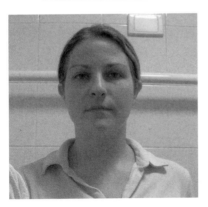

Rachael is a 30-year-old care staff member.

Introduction

- Care for older people
- Ageing population
- Dementia
- Stages of dementia
- Prevalence of dementia
- Behavioural and psychological symptoms of dementia
- Overview of the resistance to care project
- Resistance to care defined
- Resistance to care research outcome
- Resistance to care and risk of care staff injury
- References

Introduction

Care for older people

What is true for any setting is that dementia care involves intervention in some of the most personal, sensitive and private areas of people's lives, the implications of which have been raised in terms of both people with dementia[1-5] and care staff[6-14]. It is important to realise that if a person with dementia requires assistance with direct care routines they are more likely to exhibit behaviours that interfere with or prohibit care[6-9,12].

Although the evolution of approaches to dementia care in recent years[15-16] has proved beneficial to both residents and care staff, issues still exist around resistance to care that have been overlooked[17]. The stress of being involved in dementia care has been well documented. It is clearly recognised that burnout is common. Absenteeism, chronic fatigue, depression, impatience, irritability, lack of enthusiasm and physical complaints have been identified as symptoms of burnout experienced by caregivers[6,10,13,15].

This book provides practical guidelines designed to improve the interaction and outcome between the person with dementia and the care staff member, by providing strategies designed to manage, reduce or prevent resistance to care.

Ageing population

In many developed countries the population is rapidly ageing due to continuing low fertility rates and increasing longevity[18].

Developed countries show the following trends:

- 1999–2050: projected increase in older persons from 229 million in 1999 to approximately 376 million in 2050. This means that older people will account for approximately 33% of the population in developed regions of the world[18].
- By 2050, the United Nations projects that one person in every five will be aged 60 years or older[18].
- Dementia affects 1% of 65-year-olds, 40% of 85-year-olds[19] and around 50% of 95-year-olds[20].
- An estimated three quarters of a million people in the UK suffer from dementia. It is the fourth leading cause of death after heart disease, cancer and stroke[20].
- In the USA half of all care home residents suffer from Alzheimer's disease[20].

Dementia

Dementia itself is not a disease, but a condition of chronic brain failure[21], a term used to characterise a group of symptoms that accompany certain diseases[22], involving the widespread progressive decline in a range of cognitive functions that affect social, occupational and daily function[21,23]. The characteristics include 'a loss of cognitive and intellectual abilities severe enough to impair social or occupational performance' and has 'associated impairment of memory, abstract thinking, and judgement and some degree of personality change'[22].

In the elderly, dementia remains the most prevalent neuropsychiatric disorder[24]. Dementia can be classified by causes:

- Dementia in Alzheimer's disease
- Vascular dementia with Lewy bodies, frontotemporal dementia
- Other diseases, e.g. Parkinson's disease, Pick's disease, Huntington's Chorea, metabolic disorders
- Unspecified dementia

The most common causes of dementia are Alzheimer's type dementia (ATD) and vascular dementia.

Alzheimer's type dementia

This is the most common form of dementia and accounts for approximately 60% of cases. It is a progressive neurodegenerative disease[25], characterised by the slow decay of parts of the brain (cerebral atrophy). Technically the decay is due to the accumulation of tangles in the centre of brain cells and plaques outside brain cells and manifests in psychological, behavioural and physical changes to the person[25]. The progress of the disease is similar to a long slippery slope or slippery dip, characterised by three stages[26], beginning with a gradual onset, followed by a more rapid deterioration, then a slower rate of deterioration in the final phase prior to death. Caring for a person with Alzheimer's type dementia means that care staff can expect slow, reasonably predictable changes.

Vascular dementia

This is the second most common form of dementia and accounts for approximately 20% of cases. There are a number of types and causes of vascular dementia, the most common being multi-infarct dementia caused by multiple small blood vessel blockages in the brain, known as cerebrovascular accidents. These blockages result in irreversible damage to areas of the brain. It is frequently associated with high blood pressure (hypertension) as the primary cause. Vascular dementia is often described as step-like, with sudden deterioration in function followed by a plateau, that is, a period where there is no change. Caring for a person with vascular dementia means that care staff must be prepared for sudden changes. Common symptoms include, finding the person semi-conscious or unconscious, one-sided weakness causing the person to lean heavily to one side and loss of strength to the affected side of the body, facial droop and loss of speech. These symptoms may be temporary or permanent depending on the severity of the blockage.

It is important to understand that a person can have both Alzheimer's type dementia and vascular dementia, that is, they can co-exist.

Dementia with Lewy bodies

Dementia with Lewy bodies is characterised by a fluctuating course of cognitive impairment with visual or auditory hallucinations and extrapyramidal symptoms, with a slow progression to severe dementia. It is characterised by the presence of round structures called Lewy bodies that are found inside nerve cells in the cortex of the brain.

Frontotemporal dementia

This accounts for approximately 10% of cases. The diagnosis of frontotemporal dementia is based on personality changes and the atrophy of the frontal and temporal lobes of the brain. Caring for a person with frontotemporal dementia means the care staff can expect social and behavioural disinhibition, loss of social connectiveness to others, and high levels of disinterest and lack of energy.

Stages of dementia

In discussing dementia it is common to describe the person as being in a certain stage of dementia. Stages of dementia are a way of grouping aspects of function that are affected during the progress of the disease. There are a number of staging models for dementia. The benefits of staging dementia include:

- Capturing the severity and range of the dementia
- Providing a guide to the abilities of the person with dementia
- Predicting the progression of the dementia

A common staging model of Alzheimer's type dementia is made up of three stages: early stage, mild dementia; second or middle stage or moderate dementia; and third or late stage, as advanced or end stage[27]. Each stage is characterised by symptoms that assist in understanding and anticipating the presentation of the dementing process.

Stages and symptomatology of dementia

Early stage

Memory
Short term memory loss
Misplaces items
Misidentifies items
Loss of sense of direction

Cognitive ability
May not be able to do simple arithmetic
May not be able to tell the time
May lose the ability to work

Coordination – motor skills
May have slower reflexes
May not be able to drive safely

Mood and behaviour
Mood lability – mood swings
May become socially isolated
May have a flat affect
May suffer from depression or delusions

Language
May be less talkative
Expression may be vague
May have difficulty finding the right word

Ability to carry out activities of daily living
May need assistance with hygiene, dressing, grooming
May not want to bath or shower
May become incontinent

Middle stage

Memory
Short and medium term memory loss
Incapable of new memories and so cannot learn

Cognitive ability
Loss of decision-making ability
Loss of problem solving, e.g. solving jig-saw puzzles, counting
Poor judgement
Requires repeated instruction for tasks
Disorientation to time, place, person, event

Coordination – motor skills
Increased risk of falls
Disconnection between thought and action
Becomes unsteady and experiences reduction in coordination

Mood and behaviour
Labile mood – mood swings
Increasingly self-absorbed and less sensitive to others' feelings and shows little emotional warmth
Loss of understanding of relationships
May become physically restless, pacing, wandering
Suffer from delusions or hallucinations, becoming suspicious
Increasingly self-absorbed
Disrupted sleep pattern

Language
Speech slows, can be repetitive, have pauses and interruptions and have broken sentences
Loss of vocabulary, uses made-up words, sentence construction is poor
Reduction in understanding of spoken and written language

Ability to carry out activities of daily living
More dependent with hygiene, dressing, grooming
Difficulty with putting on clothes
Fear of showering
Incontinence occurs
Loss of coordinating actions for toileting, sitting and specific tasks

Last stage

Memory
Extensive memory loss

Cognitive ability
Extensive cognitive decline

Coordination – motor skills
Often unable to walk or stand by themself
Eventually may be unable to swallow

Mood and behaviour
Often become agitated
Socially withdrawn
Loss of recognition of person, place, event and time

Language
Loss of vocabulary
Echoes other people's words and repeats own words
Inability to comprehend information and instructions

Ability to carry out activities of daily living
Becomes totally dependent for all care needs

Graphic representation of the three stages of Alzheimer's disease

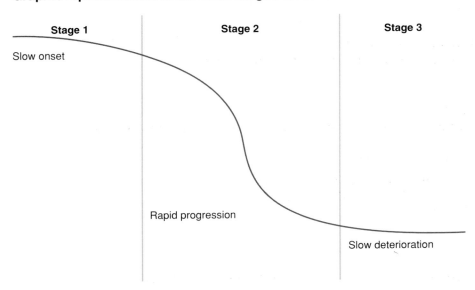

Graphic representation of vascular dementia

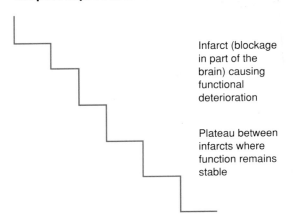

Prevalence of dementia

Much has been written discussing the prevalence of dementia and projections of dementia within the world's population. These studies all indicate an increasing prevalence paralleling the ageing population[28-34,51].

Individual country and global estimates of the prevalence of dementia and Alzheimer's type dementia (ATD), are difficult to quantify accurately. For instance, in the United States of America the estimated prevalence of persons with some form of dementia is approximated to be between 2 to 4 million[35]. A 1998 estimate of prevalence of dementia has stated that there were 18 million cases of dementia globally, with ATD afflicting approximately 5% of all persons aged over 65 years[31]. It is also estimated that 30 million people globally will suffer from ATD by 2020, with approximately 75% of cases in developing countries in Asia and Latin America[31]. These figures are consistent with other estimates[33], which indicate that by 2030 the number of ATD cases is expected to double. Alzheimer's type dementia has been described as the silent epidemic[31].

Community issue

It is not the general symptoms associated with cognitive loss in dementia that cause care staff the most distress, but the agitation that occurs in approximately 50% of persons with dementia in the middle and late stages, including behaviours of uncooperativeness, hyperactivity, disinhibition and verbal abuse[36]. Behavioural and psychological symptoms of dementia, including resistiveness and aggressive behaviours, are onerous to both families and care staff[36-41].

Admission to care homes

One of the main reasons for admission to care homes are behavioural and psychological symptoms of dementia[2,42-45], that is, the behavioural difficulties and social disruptiveness that predicates the care home admission rather than other life events[42-43,46-48].

It is not unexpected then, that behavioural and psychological symptoms, are

■ Common[49-50]
■ More severe in care homes[52] than in the wider community
■ Implicated in caregiver distress, burnout and absenteeism[17,46,52-55]

For each resident with advancing dementia accommodated in care homes there is an equivalent number residing in the community. Consequently, dementia care is a community-wide problem.

Behavioural and psychological symptoms of dementia

The main psychological symptoms are:

■ Delusions (fixed false beliefs)
■ Hallucinations (hearing or seeing something that is not there)
■ Misidentifications
■ Depressed mood
■ Anxiety

The most common forms of delusions are persecutory and paranoia[42], including the following behaviour or the belief that:

■ People are stealing their things occurs in 18–43% of patients[56]
■ The house is not their home[57]
■ The spouse is an impostor[57]
■ They have been abandoned[56]
■ Their spouse has committed infidelity[56]
■ Another person is in their house
■ Talking to a mirror as though it was another person
■ People are not who they are
■ Misidentify people on television[57]

Delusions are also identified as a significant predictor of aggression[58–59].

Catastrophic reactions are an over reaction to a minor stress and often appear in the early stages of dementia. The initial symptoms of catastrophic reactions are agitation, restlessness, such as fidgeting, facial reddening (flushing) and refusing to comply with requests or to an act, e.g. refusal to eat. These symptoms escalate to behaviours such as, yelling, screaming, pacing, banging items and posturing.

Sundowning is when the person with dementia experiences an acute increase in disorientation, deterioration in cognition, sudden onset of restlessness and confusion in the late afternoon into the early evening. It can present with an increase in resistive behaviours, delusions, disorientation and disorganisation. Often the person will have less energy for activities and demands and seem more impulsive.

Wandering is also a common behaviour in the early to middle stages of dementia.

Wandering is generally purposeful[60]. The term 'aimless' is often incorrectly applied by care staff when the person with dementia is walking with no apparent purpose or goal to the care staff member. The role of the care staff member is to identify the person's unmet needs and respond to these. One study found that 93% of journeys led to a logical destination, with 59% leading to a person or group of people, and 29% leading to a window with an outside view[61].

Purposeful wandering or walking generally has its foundations in one of the following:

■ Pre-illness habitual behaviours, such as the person who always took a walk before breakfast.
■ Long-term memory driven behaviours, e.g. taking the rubbish out.
■ The person is going somewhere or looking for something, even if we do not know what it is.
■ Delusion driven walking, such as the person who feels they are in a concentration camp or gaol.
■ Other causes, such as medical issues, e.g. pain, cerebral irritation, continence issues.

Walking is a healthy pastime and the environment should support mobility and purposeful walking (see Chapter 4, The Environment). Walking becomes problematic to care staff and others when the person with dementia:

■ Is at risk of injury
■ Is distressed
■ Is at risk of injuring others
■ Interferes with others' property

Overview of the resistance to care project

WorkCover Corporation, South Australia, identified nurses and care staff as having the highest cost injuries within specific industries in the period from 1999–2000 to 2001–2002. These were mainly caused by manual handling of patients/residents in care homes and hospitals and this rated number one for all industries. The most common hazard to care staff was found to be manual handling, followed by resistiveness and aggression.

The issue of care staff injury led to WorkCover Corporation, South Australia, funding the project 'Resistance to Care as a cause of staff injury' under the auspices of Aged and Community Services Inc. and Australian Nursing Home and Extended Care SA Inc.

The project's goal was to identify the intensity and frequency of resistive behaviours during care of the person with dementia, implement specific care interventions and then evaluate the effectiveness of these care interventions following care staff education.

Providers

- 12 sites participated
- Private/not for profit
- Inner suburbs/outer suburbs/country

Services

- Low care (hostel or assisted living) and high care (care home/nursing home)
- Mainstream and special care units (SCU)

Sample

- 249 residents' care documents were reviewed
- 5285 behavioural observations of 228 residents collected
- 400 (approximately) care staff involved

Assessment

The four variables of dementia care, the person, the care staff member, the environment and the interaction, were assessed and evaluated by:

- The review of health and socio-cultural assessments, care plans, medications
- Conducting a dementia-specific environmental audit at each site
- A three-day behavioural observation snapshot of resistance to care documented by care staff
- A care staff survey of skills, education, employment and injury history

Implementation

The evaluation led to recommendations for changes to care practices, as well as health and environmental management practices at each participating site. Education was conducted at each site, addressing the four variables.

Evaluation

Following implementation a second set of behavioural observations was repeated across the sample.

Resistance to care defined

Resistance to care is defined as

Any behavioural symptom exhibited by a person with dementia, occurring upon commencement or during care, that interferes with or prohibits care provision.

Resistance to Care Risk Rating Scale is

A four-point rating of behavioural descriptors indexed to imbue the increasing risk of care staff sustaining cumulative and/or immediate injury, as a consequence of resistance to care.

RTC Risk Rating Scale

RTC 1: Mild resistiveness	RTC 2: Semi-moderate resistiveness	RTC 3: Moderate resistiveness	RTC 4: Severe resistiveness
Agitation	Grabbing soft items, e.g. towel, clothes, face washer	Back arching	Biting
Incoherence		Chest hugging	Hitting
Indifference, not responsive to requests	Limbs and/or body going limp	Crossing limbs	Kicking
		Grabbing or holding onto carer or fixtures, e.g. chair, bed	Pinching
Mild verbal non-acceptance	Making verbal threats at normal volume		Scratching
Noisy, verbal and non-verbal	Posturing	Making verbal threats at high volume including shouting, screaming, or other strong or violent outbursts of hostility	Slapping
Passivity	Slouching into chair or bed		Striking or lashing out
Pulling away just prior to care	Spitting out, e.g. food or medication	Pulling away during care	Strong physical acts thwarting care
Not opening the mouth or swallowing	Swearing or expressing angry non-compliance	Pushing	Throwing items
Restless		Ceasing to weight bear	
Turning away or walking away	Verbally objecting to care, using words or sounds, e.g. growling	Spontaneous rigidity of body or limbs	
		Stiffening limbs	
		Waving arms and legs	

Adapted from Herz et al., 1992[62] (with thanks to the Veterans Admistration and Boston University).

Two of the descriptors 'restless' and 'agitated' have general meanings. These have been included in the RTC Risk Rating Scale as they are common terms and signal to care staff that the person is disturbed by the care activity. However, when they are used in reporting RTC behaviours, these descriptors require additional description or information. For instance, a restless episode may be further described as the resident fidgeting with the bed linen or constantly shifting position in a chair.

Resistance to care research outcome

A full report is available from the Workcover Corporation, South Australia. However, some of the key findings are summarised below.

Resistance to care episodes were recorded by direct care staff for three consecutive days at each site participating in the project. A total of 5285 behavioural observations were made by care staff of 228 residents.

Mean episode of RTC was 23.2 episodes over the period, or 7.7 episodes per day.

Moderate RTC, e.g. pushing, pulling, grabbing staff, holding solid objects, accounted for 45% of all RTC episodes. Stiffening or rigidity of limbs (n=518) was the most prevalent RTC, representing 9.8% of episodes, followed by grabbing, e.g. staff (n=351) which accounted for 6.6% of RTC episodes.

The duration of behaviour revealed that the majority of RTC persisted for 1–10 minutes, then abated.

The care activities that were associated with the most prevalent RTC were:

■ Repositioning in bed (19.4%)
■ Assisting with eating (9.5%)
■ Showering/bathing (9.3%)
■ Pad change (8.3%)
■ Dressing/undressing (8.3%)
■ Toileting (7.3%)

The most prevalent RTC behaviours were:

■ Stiffening/rigidity of limbs (moderate RTC)
■ Grabbing, including care staff (moderate RTC)
■ Confusion that occurs on commencement or during care (mild RTC)
■ Grabbing soft items (semi-moderate RTC)
■ Grabbing or holding onto fixtures (moderate RTC)
■ Agitation (mild RTC)

Duration of RTC behaviour

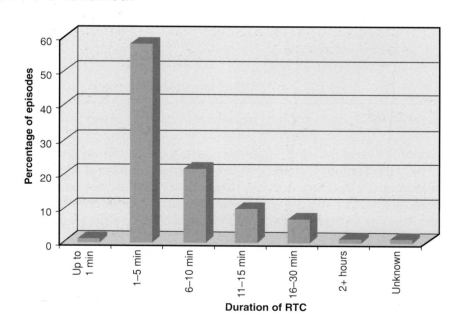

This graph shows that the majority of RTC behaviours had durations of 1–10 minutes, with 60% having a duration of 1–5 minutes and 20% having a duration of 6–10 minutes. Repeated exposure has implications in terms of cumulative injury for care staff.

Resistance to care and risk of care staff injury

Exposure to resistance to care behaviour exhibited by the older person with dementia during care activities increases the risk of care staff injury. Consequently, it is important that incidents of resistance to care are reported, and strategies implemented to prevent and manage resistance to care.

Incident and injury triangle

Underpinning care staff safety is the understanding of the relationship between the frequencies of incidents in relation to injury. Occupational health and safety investigations of care staff injuries have historically focused on the actual incident and events occurring at the time of the incident. This approach does not account for repeated minor incidents that occur in the workplace over time, which can evolve into cumulative injury. The relationship between injuries and incidents shows that for every major injury of a care staff member there are many minor incidents and injuries. By focusing on minor and significant incidents and minor injuries it is possible to reduce the chances of significant injury to care staff.

Definitions

An incident is an unforeseen event that has a risk of causing loss or injury.
Minor incident: Risk of loss or injury is low, e.g. finding water on the floor.
Major incident: Risk of loss or injury is high, e.g. slipping on spilt water but no injury.

An injury is when a person is hurt by an event.
Minor injury: A person experiences minimal harm from an event, e.g. bruising, minor sprain or strain and involves little or no lost work time.
Major injury: A person experiences major harm from an event, e.g. a major burn, prolapsed disc in the spine, involving significant lost work time.

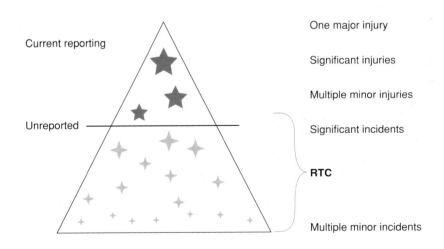

The incident and injury triangle shows that for one major injury to occur a large number of less significant injuries and incidents have occurred. Resistive behaviours generally do not immediately cause significant or major injury but can lead to cumulative injury. Therefore, by looking across all four variables, the person, the care staff, the environment and the interaction, when resistance to care occurs, it is possible to reduce care staff injuries.

The influences

There are four variables that influence the risk of RTC behaviours.
These variables are:

(1) The person (with dementia)
(2) The care staff
(3) The environment
(4) The interaction

Within these four variables are other factors that influence RTC. These are listed below, under each variable. Each variable needs to be given due consideration as to whether it impacts on the person and/or the interaction. Consequently, it is recommended that each variable and its associated profiles be reviewed to ascertain their influence. For instance, for a person who is independently mobile, issues regarding freedom of movement are paramount, in contrast to the physically dependent person whose issues may be more care staff oriented.

The person

■ Activities of daily living dependence
■ Behavioural history
■ Communication and sensory issues
■ Continence history
■ Culture and religion
■ Diagnosis, stage of dementia
■ Family involvement in care
■ Freedom of movement (restraint)
■ Gender
■ Medical assessment and review
■ Nutrition and hydration
■ Pain management
■ Psychiatric diagnosis
■ Psychotropic medications (alter thought processes, emotion, mood and behaviour)
■ Sexuality
■ Sleep

The care staff

■ Older person and dementia care experience
■ Communication skills
■ Dementia education
■ Demographic issues, e.g. cultural and social mores
■ Employment history
■ Injury profile
■ Language and discourse
■ Policy and procedures, including model of care

The environment

Physical environment

■ Orientate to the purpose of the area
■ Provide general and focal lighting for tasks
■ Include places for relaxation and stimulation
■ Occupy the person in a meaningful way
■ Encourage mobility
■ Promote independence
■ Promote a feeling of security
■ Enhance self-esteem and confidence
■ Be sensitive to each person
■ Facilitate the opportunity for family, visitors and carers to interact freely with the person

Temporal environment

■ Stability of care routines
■ Consistency of regular care staff
■ Routines promoting sleep
■ Routines promoting circadian rhythm (natural sleep/wake cycle)

The interaction

■ Continence pad change
■ Correcting sitting posture
■ Dressing
■ Assisting with eating
■ Mechanical hoist
■ Putting shoes on
■ Repositioning in bed
■ Showering/bathing
■ Stand transfer
■ Toileting
■ Transferring from lying to sitting
■ Wheelchair mobilising

References

1. Mahoney, E.K., Hurley, A.C., Volicer, L., *et al.* (1999)
   Development and testing of the Resistiveness to Care Scale. *Research in Nursing Health*, 22 (1), 27–38.
2. Kovach, C. & Meyer-Arnold, E. (1996)
   Coping with conflicting agendas: the bathing experience of cognitively impaired older adults. *Scholarly Inquiry for Nursing Practice: An International Journal*, 10 (1), 23–35.
3. Potts, H.W., Richie, M.F. & Kaas, M.J. (1996)
   Resistance to care. *Journal of Gerontological Nursing*, 22 (11), 11–16, 49–55.
4. Rabins, P.V., Mace, N.L. & Lucas, M.J. (1982)
   The impact of dementia on the family. *Journal of the American Medical Association*, 248, 333–335.
5. Devanand, D.P., Brockington, C.D., Moody, B.J., *et al.* (1992)
   Behavioural syndromes in Alzheimer's disease. *International Psychogeriatrics*, 4 (2), 161–184.
6. Beck, C.K., Baldwin, B., Modlin, T. & Lewis, S. (1990)
   Caregivers' perception of aggressive behaviour in cognitively impaired nursing home residents. *Journal of Neuroscience Nursing*, 22 (3), 169–172.
7. Burgener, S.C., Jirovec, M., Murrell, L. & Barton, D. (1992)
   Caregiver and environmental variables related to difficult behaviours in institutionalised, demented elderly persons. *Journal of Gerontology*, 47, 242–249.
8. Mistretta, E.F. & Kee, C.C. (1997)
   Caring for Alzheimer's residents in dedicated units: developing and using expertise. *Journal of Gerontological Nursing*, 19 (3), 121–126.
9. Swanson, E.A., Maas, M.L. & Buckwalter, K. (1993)
   Catastrophic reactions and other behaviours of Alzheimer's residents: special care unit compared with traditional units. *Archives of Psychiatric Nursing*, 5, 292–299.
10. Cohen-Mansfield, J. (1995)
    Assessment of disruptive behaviour/agitation in the elderly: function, methods and difficulties. *Journal of Geriatric Psychiatry Neurology*, 8 (1), 52–60.
11. Swearer, J.M. (1994)
    Behavioural disturbances in dementia. In: *Handbook of Dementing Illnesses* (ed. J.C. Morris). pp. 499–527. New York, Marcel Dekker.
12. White, M., Merrie, J. & Richie, M.F. (1996)
    Vocally disruptive behaviour. *Journal of Gerontological Nursing*, 22 (11), 23–29.
13. Andresen, G. (1995)
    Caring for People with Alzheimer's Disease: A Training Manual for Direct Care Providers. Artarmon, NSW, MacLennan & Petty Pty Ltd.
14. Burgio, L., Jones, L., Butler, F. & Engel, T. (1988)
    Behaviour problems in an urban nursing home. *Journal of Gerontology*, 14 (1), 31–34.
15. Kitwood, T. & Benson, S. (1995)
    The New Culture of Dementia Care. London, Hawker Publications.
16. Challis, D., von Abendorff, R., Brown, P. & Chesterman, J. (1996)
    Care management and dementia: an evaluation of the Lewisham intensive case management scheme. In: *Dementia: Challenges and New Directions* (ed. S. Hunter) pp. 139–164. London, Jessica Kingsley Publishers.
17. Grealy, J. & Cody, S. (2000)
    An investigation into the prevalence of resistance to care as a cause of staff injury in residential care facilities in South Australia. www.workcover.com
18. United Nations (1999)
    Population Ageing 1999. New York, Population Division. Department of Economic and Social Affairs. United Nations.
19. Bolla, L.R., Filley, C.M. & Palmer, M.R. (2000)
    Dementia DDx. Office diagnosis of the four major types of dementia. *Geriatrics*, 55 (1), 34–37.
20. Fratigilioni, L., De Ronchi, D. & Aguero-Torres, H. (1999)
    Worldwide prevalence and incidence of dementia. *Drugs, Aging*, **15** (5), 355–375.
21. McLean, S.R. (1995)
    Diagnosing dementia. In: *Dementia: A Positive View*. Canberra, Department of Veterans Affairs.
22. Kaplan, H.I. & Saddock, B.J. (1991)
    Synopsis of Psychiatry: Behavioural Sciences Clinical Psychiatry, 6th edn. Baltimore, Williams & Wilkins.
23. Strub, R.L. & Black, F.W. (1985)
    The Mental Status Examination in Neurology, 2nd edn. Sydney, F.A. Davis.
24. Bender, K. (1997)
    Article is based on the symposium, 'Agitation and aggression: Update 1997', presented at the US Psychiatric and Mental Health Congress, 14 Nov. 1997, in Orlando, Fla. *Geriatric Times*, 2 (2).

25. Cummings, J.L. (2000)
     Advances in Alzheimer's disease research: implications for new treatments. *Psychiatric Times*, 17, 1.
26. Brooks, J.O., Kraemer, H.C., Tanke, E.D. & Hachinski, V. (1993)
     The methodology of studying decline in Alzheimer's disease. *Journal of the American Geriatrics Society*, 41, 623–628.
27. Alzheimer's Association of South Australia Inc. (1999)
     Three Stages of Alzheimer's Disease. Adelaide, Alzheimer's Association of South Australia Inc.
28. Rosewarne, R. (1997)
     Care Needs of People with Dementia and Challenging Behaviour Living in Residential Facilities: Aged and Community Care Service Development and Evaluation Report 24. pp. 26–31. Canberra, Department of Health & Family Services.
29. Linderborn, K. (1988)
     The need to assess dementia. *The Journal of Gerontological Nursing*, 14 (1), 35–39.
30. Losonczy, K., White, L.R. & Brock, D.B. (1998)
     (May–June) *Prevalence and Correlates of Dementia: Survey of the Last Days of Life. Public Health Reports*, 113 (3), 273–281. US Department of Health and Human Services, USA.
31. Henderson, A.S. & Jorm, A.F. (1998)
     Dementia in Australia. Aged and Community Care Service Development and Evaluation Report. Canberra, Australian Government Printing Service.
32. Evans, D.A., Funkenstein, H.H., Albert, M.S., *et al.* (1989)
     Prevalence of Alzheimer's disease in a community population of older persons. *Journal of American Medical Association*, 262, 2551–2556.
33. Bettelheim, A. (1998)
     Alzheimer's disease: could it bankrupt the health-care system? *CQ Researcher*, 8 (19), 435–451.
34. Jorm, A.F. & Jolley, D. (1998)
     The incidence of dementia: a meta-analysis. *Neurology*, 51 (3), 156–160.
35. Hoyert, D.L. & Rosenberg, H.M. (1997)
     Alzheimer's disease as a cause of death in the United States. Public Health Report, 112, 497–505. US Department of Health and Human Services, USA.
36. McShane, E.R. (1996)
     Response to 'Coping with Conflicting Agendas: the bathing experience of cognitively impaired older adults'. *Scholarly Inquiry for Nursing Practice*, 10 (1), 37–41.
37. Burns, A. & Rabins, A. (2000)
     Carer burden in dementia. *International Journal of Geriatric Psychiatry*, 15 (1), S9–S13.
38. Donaldson, C., Tarrier, N. & Burns, A. (1997)
     The impact of the symptoms of dementia on caregivers. *British Journal of Psychiatry*, 170, 62–68.
39. Wijeratne, C. (1997)
     Pathways to morbidity in carers of dementia sufferers. *International Psychogeriatrics*, 9, 69–79.
40. Snowdon, J., Miller, R. & Vaughan, R. (1996)
     Behavioural problems in Sydney nursing homes. *International Journal of Geriatric Psychiatry*, 11, 535–541.
41. Brodaty, H., Draper, B., Saab, D. *et al.* (2001)
     Psychosis, depression and behavioural disturbances in Sydney nursing home residents: prevalence and predictors. *International Journal of Geriatric Psychiatry*, 16, 504–512.
42. Morriss, R., Rovner, B. & German, P. (1996)
     Factors contributing to nursing home admission because of disruptive behaviour. *International Journal of Geriatric Psychiatry*, 11, 243–249.
43. Pushkar Gold, D., Feldman Reis, M., Markiewicz, D. & Andres, D. (1995)
     When home caregiving ends: a longitudinal study of outcomes for caregivers of relatives with dementia. *Journal of the American Geriatrics Society*, 43, 10–16.
44. Lachs, M.S., Becker, M., Siegal, A.P., Miller, R.L. & Tinetti, M.E. (1992)
     Delusions and behavioural disturbances in cognitively impaired elderly persons. *Journal of the American Geriatric Society*, 40, 768–773.
45. Singer, C. & Bahr, A. (2005)
     Assessing and treating sleep disturbances in patients with Alzheimer's disease. *Geriatric Times*, 5, www.geriatrictimes.com/search/index.jhtml
46. Nygaard, H.A. (1991)
     Who cares for the caregiver? Factors exerting influence on nursing home admissions of demented elderly. *Scandinavian Journal of Caring Sciences*, 5 (3), 157–162.
47. Bannister, C., Ballard, C., Lana, M., Fairbairn, A. & Wilcock, G. (1998)
     (March) Placement of dementia sufferers in residential and nursing home care. *Age and Ageing*, 272, 189–194.
48. Orrell, M.W. & Bebbington, P. (1995)
     Life events and senile dementia: admission, deterioration and social environment change. *Psychological Medicine*, 25 (2), 373–386.

49. Holm, A., Michael, M., Stern, G., *et al.* (1999)
The outcomes of an inpatient program for geriatric patients with dementia and dysfunctional behaviours. *Gerontologist*, 39 (6), 668–676.

50. Cohen-Mansfield, J., Marx, M.S., Werner, P. & Lipson, S. (1993)
Assessment and management of behaviour problems in the nursing home setting. In: *Improving Care in the Nursing Home: Comprehensive Reviews of Clinical Research* (eds L. Z. Rubenstein & D. Wieland). London, Sage Publications.

51. Ray, W., Taylor, J., Lichtenstein. & Meador, G. (1992)
The Nursing Home Behaviour Problem Scale. *Journal of Gerontology*, 47 (1), M9–16.

52. Hallberg, I. & Norberg, A. (1995)
Nurses' experience of strain and their reactions in the care of severely demented patients. *International Journal of Geriatric Psychiatry*, 10, 757–766.

53. Wood, S., Cummings, J., Barclay, T., Hsu, M., Allahyar, M. & Schnelle, J. (1999)
Assessing the impact of neuropsychiatric symptoms on distress in professional caregivers. *Ageing and Mental Health*, 3, 241–245.

54. Zanetti, O., Magni, E., Sandri, C., Frisoni, G.B., Bianchetti, A. & Trabucchi, M. (1996)
Determinants of burden in an Italian sample of Alzheimer's patient caregivers. *Journal of Cross-cultural Gerontology*, 11, 17–27.

55. Rosewarne, R. (1997)
Care Needs of People with Dementia and Challenging Behaviour Living in Residential Facilities: Aged and Community Care Service Development and Evaluation Reports 24. pp. 26–31. Canberra, Department of Health & Family Services.

56. Tariot, P.N. & Blazina, L. (1993)
The psychopathology of dementia. In: *Handbook of Dementing Illness* (ed. J. Morris). New York, Marcel Dekker.

57. Mireas, A. & Cummings, J. (2000)
In: *Dementia* (eds J. O'Brien, D. Ames & A. Burns), 2nd edn. New York, Arnold.

58. Deutsch, L.H., Bylsma, F.W., Rovner, B.W., Steele, C. & Folstein, M.F. (1991)
Psychosis and physical aggression in probable Alzheimer's disease. *American Journal of Psychiatry*, 148, 1159–1163.

59. Gilley, D.W., Wilson, R.S., Beckett, L.A. & Evans, D.A. (1997)
Psychotic symptoms and physically aggressive behaviour in Alzheimer's disease. *Journal of the American Geriatric Society*, 45, 1074–1079.

60. McGregor, I. & Bell, J. (1994)
Buzzing with life, energy and drive. *Journal of Dementia Care*, 2 (6), 20–21.

61. Hussein, R. (1982)
Stimulus control in modification of problematic behaviour in elderly institutionalised patients. *International Journal of Behavioural Geriatrics*, 1 (33), 42.

62. Herz, L.R., Volicer, L., Ross, V. & Rheaume, Y. (1992)
A single case study method for treating resistiveness in patients with Alzheimer's disease. *Hospital and Community Psychiatry*, 437.

1 The Person

- Ageing
- Movement
- Visual field/spatial perception
- Reflexes
- Profiling the person
- Restraint
- Continence guidelines
- References

1 The Person

Ageing

Most older persons have active lives, and life is just as rewarding, interesting and diverse as at any other time in their life. However, for some older people the ageing process can feel as though it is marked by functional losses, such as:

- Physical changes
- Sensory changes
- Cognitive changes

Individually, or in combination, these changes can lead to the need for care.

The three aims of this section are:

(1) To introduce care staff to concepts of change as part of the ageing process.
(2) To increase care staff understanding of the impact that each change can have on an older person.
(3) To begin to show how a care staff member can compensate, to some degree, for these changes.

What we do know is that the greater the number of changes experienced by the older person, the more dependent the person becomes on care staff to meet their needs. Therefore, the greater the cognitive loss the more personal the nature of care becomes, so there is greater likelihood of resistance to care.

Physical changes
+
Sensory changes
+
Cognitive changes
=
Increasing risk of RTC

This chapter of the book is comprised of six subsections:

(1) Movement
(2) Spatial perception (interpretation of space, depth, light, colour, contrast, angles and objects in relation to the position of the person)
(3) Use of reflexes to elicit purposeful movement
(4) Profiling the person
(5) Restraint
(6) Continence guidelines

Movement

Movement explores the reduced mechanical and sensory changes that take place as part of the ageing process. This includes, but is not limited to:

■ Range of motion, that is, movement at the joints.
■ Muscle strength that enables limbs to move.
■ Sensation, the ability to feel touch.
■ Endurance, the ability to do a task without getting tired.

Why is this important?

At times the older person with dementia has to be assisted with body movements, ranging from verbal or physical prompts to being fully assisted. If the care staff member is unaware of the person's mechanical or sensory limitations then he/she might place a glass of juice out of reach or ask the person to brush their hair when they cannot reach their head, or get the person to sit in a chair that is too low, making it difficult to sit down and very difficult to get up out of the chair. These situations are likely to cause the older person frustration, and for a person with dementia who doesn't know their own limitations, an injury.

The care staff member then needs to be aware that:

(1) The older person may not have normal range of movement, strength, sensation or endurance.
(2) A change or loss in any one of these areas will affect function. Even simple tasks may be affected, such as reaching for a glass of juice or being able to brush their hair.

So how far can you move a limb or a joint?

Often a physiotherapist or occupational therapist will undertake a movement analysis on an older person, that is, work out what is required to undertake a certain activity. However, where this has not happened it is important to remember the following:

(1) Think how far you can move one of your joints or limbs; for the older person it will be less.
(2) Be careful not to move the joint beyond the person's ability.
(3) In most cases, at the end of a person's full extension, you will start feeling an increasing resistance, that is, it will take more pressure from you to keep going. This means that you have reached the maximum movement – STOP. Any further pressure may cause injury. However, sometimes there is no resistance from the person's muscles, e.g. following a stroke (cerebrovascular accident) that leads to muscle wasting in the shoulder and so the arm may seem floppy. You must be very careful in this situation and a health professional should provide guidelines on range of movement.

Terminology

In this book, specific terms are used to describe Molly (the person with dementia) and Angela's (care staff member) movements. The aim is to familiarise care staff with the main concepts of movement rather than detailed biomechanics, so only a limited number of the main movements are used.

(1) Degrees

Health professionals use degrees to describe the range of movement of a body part. For instance, how far the head can turn from looking straight ahead (0°) to looking over your shoulder (about 90°). This movement is called neck rotation. The elbow has a much greater degree of movement and can be fully flexed or bent (0°) to being fully extended or straightened (about 150°).

Degrees is a measure of angles.

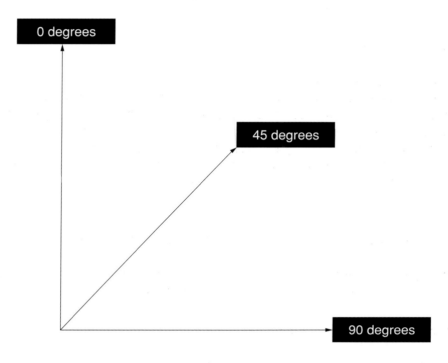

(2) Joint movements

  (a) Rotation
  (b) Extension and flexion
  (c) Abduction and adduction

(a) Rotation

Neck rotation is measured from the point of the face being directly forward, then turning the face to the left or right. An adult should have approximately 90° neck rotation, that is, from looking directly forward to turning the head as far as possible to the right. Consequently, less than 45° is considered to be a reduced or limited neck rotation.

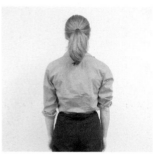

0° neck rotation.

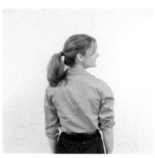

90° neck rotation.

(b) Extension and flexion

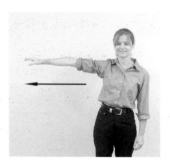

Extension is the term used to describe where a limb is made straight, or where the two ends of any jointed part are moved away from each other.

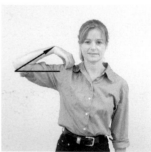

Flexion is the opposite of extension, where the limb is bent, or when the two ends of any jointed part are moved toward each other.

(c) Abduction and adduction

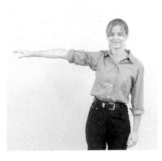

Abduction is where a limb is moved away from the body or midline.

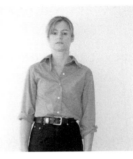

Adduction is the opposite of abduction, where a limb is moved toward the body or midline.

(3) Functional range of movement

Functional range of movement is the movement of a joint, or combination of joints, that is required to perform a specific task. For example, putting shoes on requires quite different body movements than reaching for a cup off a shelf above head height.

Functional movements usually appear as a diagonal pattern[1].

■ Swinging arms during walking move in a diagonal pattern across the front of the body.
■ The hand moves in diagonal pattern from the side of the body to reach for a cup placed on a table in front of the person.

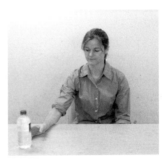

Placing an item outside the diagonal pattern, away from the centre of the body, makes it difficult to reach.

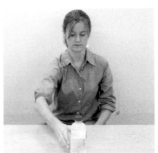

It is generally easier for a person to reach items centred directly in front of them.

Ageing and movement

Secondary to the ageing process, there is often injury and/or chronic disease.

- Presence of pain
- Depression
- Decreased muscle strength
- Soft tissue/bone injury and degeneration
- Sensory changes in hearing, sight, touch and taste

The presence of any one or more of these factors in association with any physical, cognitive or sensory change can impair function. This impairment often presents as a reduced ability to perform activities of daily living, which then leads to a dependency on care staff to help with their needs.

The physical changes in ageing that lead to an older person requiring care are presented in this section by contrasting:

- Angela, a fit and able adult, with
- Molly, a person with dementia who requires daily assistance with activities of daily living

When looking at the photos note Molly's reduced range of movement compared to Angela.

Posture, balance and trunk rotation

Standing posture affects many aspects of a person's ability to stand and walk, as well as the speed at which a person can adjust to see short, medium and long distances. In these photos the effect of posture on visual field is shown.

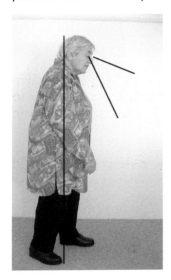

Molly can only see a short distance in front of her and has great difficulty seeing anything at head height or higher.

Molly will need to change her posture by stopping and leaning back to see medium to long distances in front or above her.

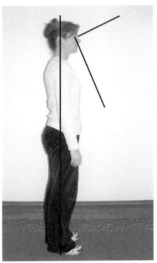

Angela can see downwards, directly in front, side to side and above her head without significantly changing her posture.

✓ **Key Learning:**   Unless you are diagonally in front and at close range the person may not know you are there, because their visual field is narrow.

Neck rotation

A reduction in neck rotation in the person can result in a number of changes, such as a narrowing of their visual field and an altered spatial perception.

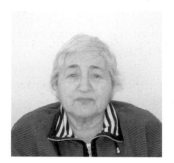

0° neck rotation.

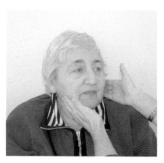

Approximately 0–40° neck rotation. With a potentially limited range of neck movement the scope of area that Molly is able to visually scan and attend is significantly reduced.

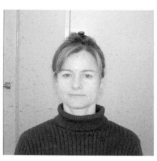

0° neck rotation.

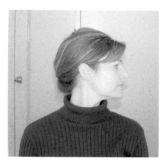

Angela can rotate her neck the full 90° without changing her posture.

✓ **Key Learning:**   Being diagonally in front of the person means you should stand where the older person need only turn their head (neck rotation) and not move any other part of their body to see you.

Posture and walking

Walking is natural for most people. Little thought is given to walking until an event occurs that impacts on walking, from stubbing one's toe, breaking a bone in a leg, or walking on a hot surface.

For the older person, walking can be both challenging and sometimes risky. In this first photograph we illustrate some of the mechanisms of walking.

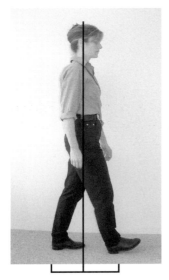

When Angela walks her upper body, and therefore most of her weight, is centred equally over her hips and is equally distributed across both feet.

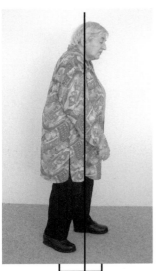

When Molly walks notice that her weight is not centred over her hips, but is centred over her front left foot rather than equally distributed across her two feet.

Consequently, Molly is at greater risk of tripping and if she loses her balance she has a greater tendency to fall forward.

✓ **Key Learning:**   Allow the older person time to maintain and correct their balance. The older person may need to stop and balance before interacting.

Posture and walking (with walking frame)

In these photographs the effect of posture on visual field when walking with a walking frame is shown.

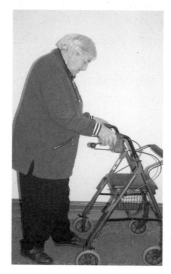

Molly can only see a short distance in front of her and has great difficulty seeing anything directly in front at head height or higher.

Molly will need to change her posture to see directly in front or above her.

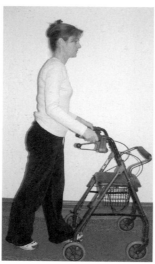

Angela can see both downwards, directly in front and above her head without changing her posture.

✓ **Key Learning:**   The older person may need to stop walking with their frame and balance before interacting.

Posture and walking (with walking frame)

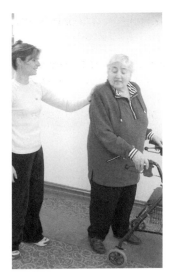

Molly does not know that Angela has come up from behind until Angela touches Molly on the shoulder. Molly has limited range of movement in her trunk so she has to stop, gain her balance, then turn around.

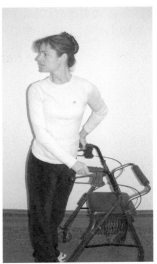

This contrasts with Angela's full range of movement that allows her to maintain the direction of her feet and turn to look behind her.

✓ **Key Learning:**   Walk past the person and position yourself inside their visual field before interacting. Try not to approach them from behind as they may not know you are there.

Posture and walking (approaching from behind)

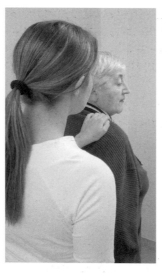

The photograph on the left depicts Molly's view when she turns to look over her shoulder. Molly's limited neck and trunk rotation means she can only see Rachael's shirt and waist.

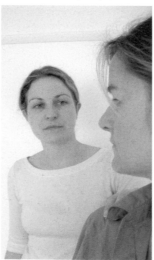

On the other hand, because Angela has full neck and trunk rotation she can turn and see that Rachael is standing behind or beside her.

✓ **Key Learning:**   A person with dementia may not recognise events or persons outside their visual field and so do not know you are there until you touch them on the shoulder, which may frighten them.

Shoulder, elbow, wrist and hand range of movement

We often take for granted the functions associated with the shoulder, elbow and hand, such as reaching up to get something out of a cupboard, brushing our hair or holding a utensil. Molly finds many simple tasks difficult, such as brushing her hair, pulling a top over her head, bringing food up to her mouth, fastening and unfastening a bra and reaching for a cup, due to reduced function in her shoulders, elbows, wrists and hands.

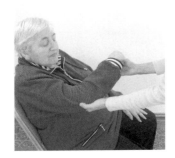

Molly has reduced range of movement in her shoulder and elbow. This results in Molly having difficulty performing the required action, such as reaching items that are not in her functional range of movement.

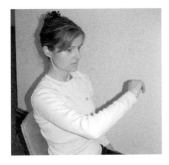

Angela has full range of movement in her shoulder and elbow.

✓ **Key Learning:**   Items placed in front of an older person need to be centred in front of them.

Shoulder, elbow, wrist and hand range of movement

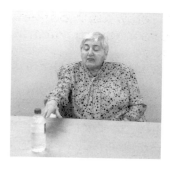

Placing an object, such as a glass, out to the right side of the table setting makes it difficult for Molly to pick it up.

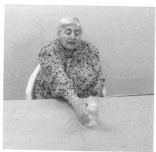

On the other hand, by placing the glass within Molly's functional range of movement promotes her independence, as she can easily reach and pick it up.

✓ **Key Learning:**   Promote independence by placing items on tables centred in front of the older person.

Shoulder, elbow, wrist and hand range of movement

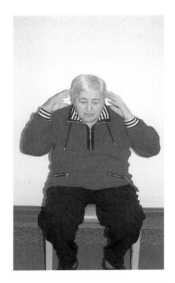

To raise her arms above her shoulders, Molly needs to compensate by trunk and neck flexion, that is, she has to lean forward. To push her arms further might elicit pain or injury.

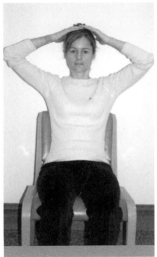

Notice that Angela maintains her balance and places her hands on her head quite easily.

| ✓ **Key Learning:** | Encourage the older person to self-care, e.g. brush own hair, then assist with completion of care when the older person does not have the range of movement to enable them to perform other care activities. Undertake proper range of movement assessment to determine an older person's care needs and don't have unrealistic expectations. |

Hand range of movement

In the ageing process, injury and/or chronic disease may also affect the hand. This is seen as a reduced ability to grasp and release and manipulate objects necessary for daily function. This is illustrated in the following examples, comparing Angela's normal adult hand and Molly's ageing hand.

Often, with loss of range of movement, there is:

- Presence of pain
- Decreased muscle strength
- Soft tissue or bone degeneration

These can lead to impaired hand function including:

- Reduced ability to grasp
- Reduced ability to manipulate small objects

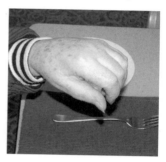

Note the swollen joints (in this case related to arthritis) in Molly's hand.

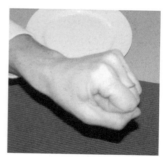

Contrast this with Angela's hand that has fine joints and no swelling, giving her full range of movement.

✓ **Key Learning:**   In the older person, swollen joints can be painful and reduce range of movement and fine motor skills.

The hand range of movement

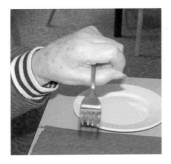

To compensate for the reduced range of movement of Molly's fingers, it may be appropriate to supply her with adapted cutlery. Larger cylindrical handles reduce the force required of the musculature of the hand, making it easier for Molly to grip the utensil.

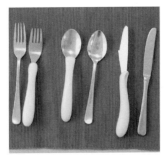

Comparison of normal cutlery handle with adapted cutlery. Adaptive cutlery reduces the amount of force required by finger and hand muscles to grip the cutlery.

✓ **Key Learning:** To maintain independence with an activity of daily living, the older person may need to change their approach to the activity, e.g. the way they hold cutlery may need to be different, or the utensils used may need to be modified.

The hand range of movement

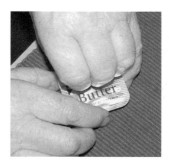

People in care homes and hospitals are often provided with individual servings of condiments, including butter, margarine and jams, for food safety reasons.

Molly lacks the fine motor movements and flexibility of finger movement required to lift the lid.

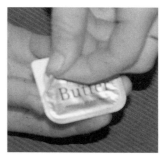

Angela's fingers have the fine motor coordination to lift the lid easily.

✓ **Key Learning:**   Assess the older person for fine motor movement dexterity and then assess each activity of daily living to determine if other strategies need to be put in place to keep the older person independent.

Lower body movements involving the hips, knees and feet

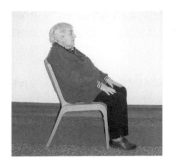

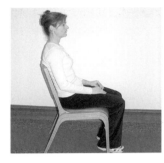

In these photographs the effect of posture on sitting position is shown. Although Molly and Angela appear to have the same sitting posture there are slight but important differences.

Molly's weight is positioned further back into the chair compared to Angela; therefore repositioning her would be more difficult.

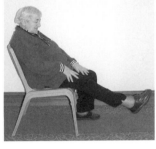

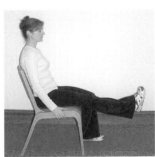

These two photographs highlight the difference in leg extension and upper leg strength between Molly and Angela.

Molly has reduced hip and knee extension and flexion compared with Angela.

✓ **Key Learning:**   Assess the older person for balance, ability to maintain balance and lower body strength, for activities such as sitting in a chair, repositioning in a chair and ability to stand up from a sitting position.

Upper and lower body range of movement

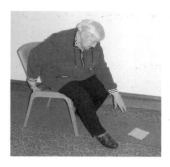

These photographs show the effect of reduced range of movement in Molly's trunk and limbs, and reduced sitting balance when leaning forward.

When leaning forward notice how Molly has stabilised herself by holding the side of the chair, due to reduced range of movement of her trunk and hips. If she did not, she would have overbalanced and fallen forward.

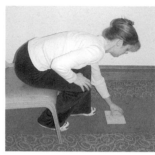

This contrasts with Angela's ability to simply lean forward, counter-balancing her position with her left foot, enabling her to reach the serviette easily.

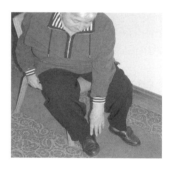

Molly has reduced range of movement in her hips, knees and ankles, which prevents her from raising her leg.

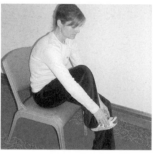

This contrasts with Angela who can easily raise and cross her leg. Notice that she does not need to bend forward or counter-balance herself to do this.

✓ **Key Learning:**   Assistive devices can promote independence and reduce the risk of falls.

Visual field/spatial perception

In persons with dementia, sensory changes can impact significantly on their ability to sense, interpret and respond to the environment.

Spatial perception is concerned with the older person's interpretation of space, depth, height, colour, contrast, angles and objects in relation to their position within their environment, and so defining the environment becomes increasingly important. This can be achieved with the use of lighting, colour contrast and signs or symbols.

What we can see, hear, smell and touch determines our view of the world and our relationship to it, such as:

■ Time of day
■ Events happening around us
■ Our role in the events happening around us
■ Whether we are safe or in danger

Therefore, as dementia progresses the person may need more cues to understand and interact with the environment and with others. Three examples of this are given below. Refer to the Environment chapter for a more detailed coverage of this topic.

Spatial perception at meals

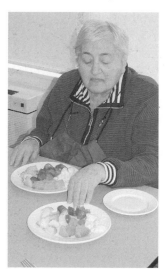

Molly is unable to distinguish her personal space and so takes food from both plates on the table.

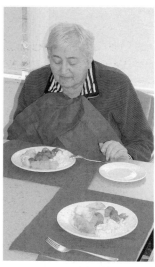

Placing a contrasting coloured placemat under Molly's plate helps define what is hers. Molly will then only eat from her plate.

✓ **Key Learning:**   Once the plated food is further defined by contrasting coloured placemats Molly confines herself to her own food.

Spatial perception for a person who has had a cerebrovascular accident (CVA or stroke)

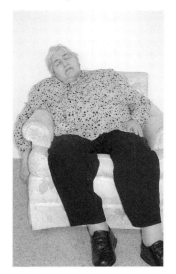

Molly has had a left CVA, causing right-sided weakness. This causes Molly to lean heavily to her right side. When Molly is leaning to the right her spatial perception is of two care staff standing upright.

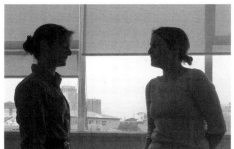

When Rachael attempts to correct Molly's sitting position quickly it feels to Molly as though she is being positioned at the wrong angle. In an upright position Molly's spatial perception is of the two care staff members standing diagonally.

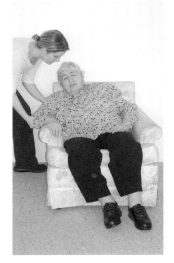

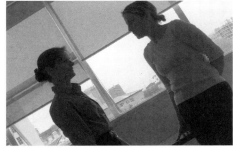

Consequently, Molly resists the correction by leaning more heavily to the right in an attempt to maintain her posture, and correct her spatial perception.

✓ **Key Learning:** Molly needs to be upright for correct posture, which prevents back and neck ache, and potential contractures. However, be aware that in the upright position Molly's spatial perception will be skewed to the left or right immediately following a correction in her posture.

Spatial perception and lighting

In this photograph two care staff are standing in front of west facing windows in the afternoon.

The glare affects Molly's vision, resulting in Molly being able to see the dark outline of the two care staff members but not who they are.

Consequently, the care staff might be viewed as strangers and if they commence care without engaging Molly first she may get a fright and respond with resistance to care.

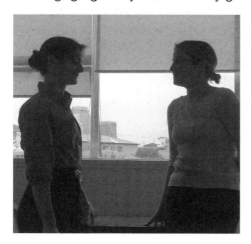

✓ **Key Learning:**   Be aware that strong lighting or sunlight glare behind you may reduce the older person's ability to see you clearly.

Reflexes

Use of reflexes to elicit purposeful movement

At birth the brain is not fully developed and so we are born with innate reflexes, that is, basic, involuntary and simple reflexes that serve to prevent harm while the brain is maturing. As the brain matures it modifies or extinguishes these reflexes. Our ability to walk and move quickly out of harm's way are built on these reflexes. These reflexes slowly disappear from six months of age and then fully disappear by eighteen months of age. Some, or all, of these reflexes often reappear in adults who have suffered a brain injury, e.g. from a motor vehicle accident or cerebrovascular accident. Although not well documented, these reflexes often reappear in people with advancing dementia. This section deals specifically with six reflexes (listed below), and how to stimulate them to elicit five different responses that assist with care delivery. These techniques are then incorporated into the Interaction chapter of the book.

(1) The Hand: stimulating grasping (part A and B): the grasp reflex
(2) The Hand: releasing the grip (part A and B): the placing reaction of the upper limb leads to the opening of the hand
(3) Decreasing the level of arousal and agitation: tactile input over the sensory distribution of the back (posterior rami)
(4) Rooting reflex: assisting to eat
(5) Suck reflex: assisting to eat
(6) Withdrawal reflex: kicking action

The hand: stimulating grasp reflex (part A)

Description
The grasp reflex is where the hand curls into a fist.
This usually happens spontaneously when an object is placed in a person's hand.

Aim
To elicit a grasping reflex around a utensil, e.g. spoon.

Procedure
Stimulate the palm of the hand.
The person then grasps the object and it is often difficult to remove the object from the person's hand.

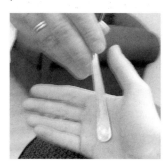

(1) Stimulation of the palm with the spoon.

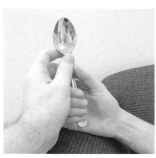

(2) Further assistance with the grasping reflex by gently closing the hand around the spoon.

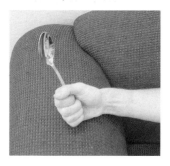

(3) Full grasp of spoon.

✓ **Key Learning:**   Support the procedure by using key words, verbal prompts and, if required, some physical assistance.

The hand: stimulating grasp reflex (part B)

Description
The grasp reflex is where the hand curls into a fist.
This is usually seen when an object is placed in a person's hand.

Aim
To elicit a grasping reflex.

Procedure
The grasp reflex is achieved by stimulating the interior aspect of the forearm with cotton wool, tissue or similar soft material.

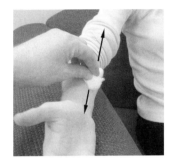 (1) Stimulation of the inside of the arm with tissue or cotton wool.

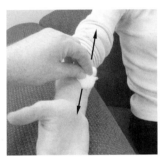 (2) Gently stroke the inside of the arm.

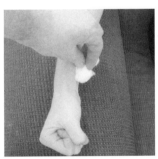 (3) The stimulation leads to the closing of the hand curling into a fist.

✓ **Key Learning:**   Stroking should be very light, like butterfly wings touching the skin.

The hand: releasing the grasp reflex/grip (A)

Description
Releasing the grasp reflex is where the hand uncurls from a fist to an open hand.
This is usually seen when you want to release an object.

Aim
To stimulate a release of the object being held.

Procedure
Lightly stroke the back of the person's hand, top and length of the forearm with cotton wool, tissue or similar soft material.
The relaxation of the fist or grasp is achieved by stimulating the extensor muscles of the hand.

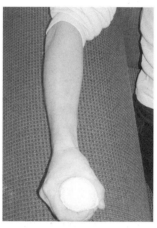

1. Note firm hold of the object.

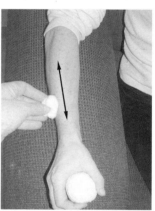

2. Lightly brush the top and length of the forearm. (Stimulation of extensor muscles).

    The brushing of the skin should be as light as butterfly wings.

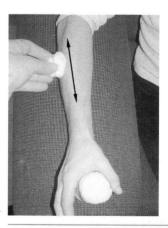

3. Eventual release of the object.

✓ **Key Learning:**   The stroking should be very light, like butterfly wings touching the skin.

The hand: releasing the grasp reflex/grip (B)

Description
Releasing the grasp reflex is where the hand uncurls from a fist to an open hand.
This is usually seen when you want to release an object.

Aim
To stimulate a release of the object being held.

Procedure
Lightly stroke the back of the hand.
The relaxation of the fist or grasp is achieved by stimulating the extensor muscles of the hand.

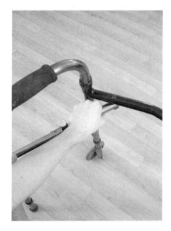

(1) Tight clasping of the lower rail of the walking frame.

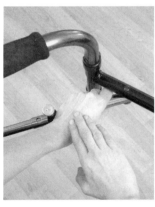

(2) Gentle, light stroking of the back of the hand, using finger tips, cotton wool or tissue.

The touch of the skin should feel like butterfly wings.

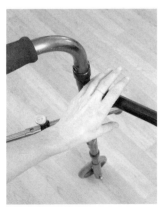

(3) Grip released.

✓ **Key Learning:**   Support the process by using key words, verbal prompts and, if required, some physical assistance.

Decreasing the level of arousal and agitation

Description
Tactile input over the sensory distribution of the back (posterior rami) leads to a calming effect through an inhibitory effect on the sympathetic chain of the autonomic nervous system.

Aim
To induce relaxation.

Procedure
Preferably perform in a quiet environment.
Place the person in a prone or sidelying (coma) position, although it can be performed in a sitting position as illustrated.
The care staff's hand firmly strokes the person's back alongside the spine, from the base of neck to below the hips in a slow rhythmic manner.

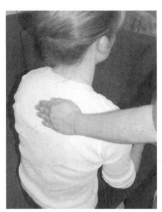

Stroke up and down in rhythmic movement from just below the hips to the nape of the neck.

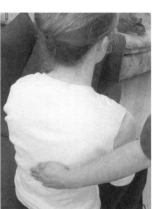

Most effective in a quieter environment.

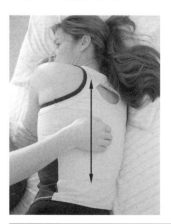

Relaxation will be shown by slowed breathing, less muscle tension and less talking.

✓ **Key Learning:**   It is preferable to reduce background noise and ensure the room is a comfortable temperature.

Rooting reflex: assisting to eat

Description
Tactile stimulation of the cheek to elicit the rooting response leading to opening of the mouth.

Aim
To stimulate the opening of the mouth and acceptance of the food.

Procedure
Preferably perform in a quiet environment.

Gently stroke the person's cheek using the back of a finger, or cotton wool, or a very soft item, to give the sensation of butterfly wings touching the skin.

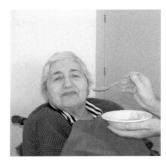

In this photograph Molly's head is turned away from the food being offered.

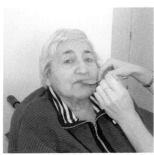

In this photograph the care staff member gently strokes Molly's left cheek with the back of her finger (cotton wool could also be used), which turns Molly's face towards the spoon placed against her lips.

✓ **Key Learning:**   Recommended to be performed simultaneously with the suck reflex.

Suck reflex: assisting to eat

Description
Tactile stimulation of the upper lip to elicit the root response.

Aim
To stimulate Molly to face the food and open her mouth to accept the food.

Procedure
Preferably perform in a quiet environment.
Gently stroke the person's upper lip with a finger, and/or place (smear) a small amount of the food on the upper lip.

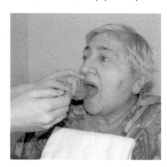

Stimulation of top lip leads to mouth opening.

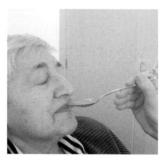

Place (smear) some food on to the top lip so Molly elicits the root response and opens her mouth and licks the food off her upper lip.

✓ **Key Learning:** Recommended to be performed simultaneously with the rooting reflex.

Withdrawal reflex: kick action

Description
Tactile stimulation of the underside of the foot can elicit a kicking action, that is, moving the foot away from the irritating stimuli. This reflex is based on a protective, safety response to potential harm of the foot.

Aim
To stimulate the kicking reflex to get Molly to uncross her legs.

Procedure
Molly cannot understand that Rachael wants Molly's legs uncrossed, so rather than pulling the legs apart Rachael uses the withdrawal reflex. Preferably perform in a quiet environment. Stand on one side:

■ With one hand: gently tickle the underside of Molly's foot (plantar aspect) with a finger. If this does not elicit a response replace with firm strokes.
■ With the other hand: hold the ankle or calf of the upper foot to guide it away from you.

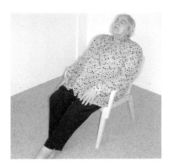

Molly has crossed her legs and her body and legs are rigid.

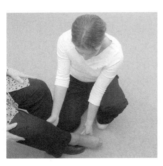

Rachael gently tickles the underside of Molly's foot.

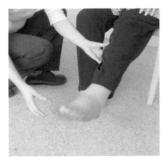

Molly responds to the tickle or stroke by eliciting the withdrawal reflex. Her legs are now uncrossed.

✓ **Key Learning:** This technique should be performed from the opposite side of which the uppermost leg is crossed. If the left leg is crossed over the right leg then squat to the right side. In this position you are less likely to be kicked. This technique should not be performed on a person who has existing spasticity of the leg.

Profiling the person

This section provides an overview of some of the key issues that should be taken into account when assessing the person with dementia.

Gender

■ Language
Males in the early and middle stages of ATD tend to retain their verbal skills longer than females[2-3].

■ Behaviour
Females with ATD tend to be more reclusive and emotionally labile[4]. Males have been found to exhibit greater problem behaviours, such as wandering, aggressiveness and socially inappropriate behaviour, in the advanced stages of ATD[5-6].

Culture

■ In select cultures aged care placement of a relative is perceived as abandoning the person[7].

■ The person with dementia often reverts to their primary language.

■ The person with dementia who has learnt English as a second language may be unfamiliar with health care terms.

■ Family interviews are important as they help obtain information on the person's history, such as their eating and toileting routines, expression of pain, and social needs.

Spiritual/religious considerations

■ Spiritual expression and religious rites can be a significant defining characteristic of the person. Spiritual beliefs and practices are often embedded from early childhood and develop over a lifetime. Consequently, spirituality can influence the person's self-expression; such as in relationships, expressed values, and in defining the person's meaning in life.

■ As dementia progresses the person may no longer be able to outwardly express their spiritual needs in a meaningful way, thus becoming reliant upon care staff. Consequently, insight into the person can also require understanding of the person's spiritual self, an issue that must be addressed with sensitivity and openness, and incorporated into care. Discussion with the person, as well as gathering information about past spiritual, cultural and religious practice from family and friends, may help in offering meaningful choices which respect the 'whole' person.

■ Pastoral care is an integral part of dementia care, for the person with dementia, and also the care staff, and can facilitate greater meaning to the care of the person with dementia, as well as meeting the person's spiritual needs. Consulting with a trained, skilled pastoral care practitioner will assist in offering appropriate suggestions for ongoing spiritual nurture that are consistent with the person's expressed spirituality.

Sexuality

■ Our immediate understanding of a person's sexuality is often through the observation of the person. This may include observation of the person's type and style of clothing (both present and as depicted in photographs from earlier life), movement, relationship structures, sexual relations, current or historical employment and expressed values.

■ The person with dementia may no longer be able to actively determine or control the expression of their sexuality in a way that they have been accustomed. For instance, the person may no longer be able to actively choose their clothing, meals and friends, due to loss of cognition and care staff choice.

■ The last bastion of sexual identity can be clothing choice, use of preferred name and opportunities to meaningfully interact on an individual level, including touch. Care staff can begin facilitating the expression of the person's sexuality by focusing on these three factors.

Communication and sensory issues

■ Care staff need to be skilled communicators because it influences the behaviour of the person with dementia[8].
■ Care staff who show a relaxed and calm approach have a calming influence upon the person with dementia[9].
■ Sensory impairment or loss can be a significant contributor to behavioural disturbance.
■ It is important to regularly assess the person for sensory changes and ensure that they have functioning hearing aids and appropriate eye glasses[10–11].

Medical assessment and review

■ Acute illness, such as a urinary tract infection can cause a sudden change in behaviour.
■ A long-term condition, such as arthritis, can also cause behaviour to modify over time.
■ A mental status examination establishes the level of cognitive functioning and can assist in the development of care plans.

Dementia diagnosis

■ Different causes of dementia determine prognosis, treatment and behaviour[12].
■ Stage of dementia is an important indicator of potential behavioural disturbance as behaviours worsen in the second and third stages of dementia, paralleling the cognitive decline[13–14].
■ If the dementia affects the frontal lobe of the brain, the person may not understand what is socially appropriate. This person may exhibit impulsive behaviours, such as yelling and sexually inappropriate behaviours.

Psychiatric diagnosis

■ Symptoms of psychiatric illnesses can still appear during dementia, e.g. delusions and hallucinations in schizophrenia[15].

■ Depression is common in people with dementia[12,16] and ranges from 42% in care home persons to an estimated 86%[17].

■ Diagnosing depression in dementia can be quite complex, due to similarity of presenting symptoms[16,18–19].

■ Depression is commonly associated with increased difficulties in communication and activities of daily living dependence.

■ Presenting symptoms of depression frequently relate to inner feelings such as anxiety, flat mood, disinterest, helplessness, hopelessness and worthlessness[12].

Medication

■ Polypharmacy (administration of a number of different medications) is indicated as a cause of agitation[14].

■ There is also concern regarding the use of typical antipsychotic medication, due to their side effect profile, including tardive dyskinesia, anticholinergic toxicity, postural hypotension and sedation[20–23].

■ Benzodiazepines can exacerbate apraxia, disorientation, confusion, and can cause psychomotor impairment[24].

■ Benzodiazepines have implications in falls[12,25].

■ Benzodiazepines can be appropriate in the management of 'anxiety and insomnia in the absence of psychotic features'[25].

Behaviours

■ Often the person with dementia will exhibit more than one behaviour that care staff find challenging, e.g. verbal disruption, aggression, wandering[26].

Hygiene care

■ The severity of behavioural and psychological symptoms of dementia increases during interventions in personal hygiene and other direct care activities[27–31]. Consequently, it is important to modify care based on the person's needs, in consideration of their behaviour.

Pain assessment

■ Age related chronic pain conditions, such as neuralgia and osteoarthritis, can be exacerbated by a sedentary lifestyle[32].

■ There is an increase in the prevalence of pain with ageing[30,32–33].

■ Pain in care home (nursing home) populations ranges from 45% to 80%[30].

■ Pain episodes can manifest as disturbed behaviours in people with cognitive deficits[33–35].

Sleep

■ A person-oriented approach to care can reduce agitation and improve 24-hour sleep patterns in persons with dementia in a care home[9].
■ Both physical discomfort and sleep deprivation are contributors to agitated behaviour[36].
■ It is important to establish a sleep pattern and develop a routine toward settling.
■ If insomnia is experienced consider reducing daytime naps, increase daytime exercise and/or assess for medical causes.

Nutrition and hydration

■ Dehydration can increase irritability, reduce the ability to concentrate and contribute to ill-health, e.g. urinary tract infections or constipation.
■ Hunger can increase agitation.
■ Malnourishment can reduce a person's capacity to undertake activities of daily living.
■ Poor oral intake can be related to mouth ulcers, ill-fitting dentures, swallowing difficulties, change in medication, or unfamiliar food.

Restraint

Restraint is any action which restricts the physical and/or psychological freedom of the person in a negative sense[37].

The rule of thumb to determine if an action is considered restraint.

(1) Does the object restrict the person's free movement?
(2) Is it, at least, difficult for the person to remove the object?

Yes to both indicates restraint[38].

Reasons for restraint:

■ Safety
■ Policy permitting use of restraint
■ Maintenance of medical treatment
■ Care staff protection
■ Care staff's own sense of security and comfort
■ Legal liability
■ Behaviour management

Those generally restrained:

■ Advanced age
■ Cognitively impaired
■ Visually impaired
■ History of falling
■ Agitated
■ Have behaviours such as:
    ■ verbal and physical aggressiveness
    ■ resistance to treatments and care
    ■ restlessness and confusion
    ■ wandering
    ■ disruptive behaviour

Consequences of restraint[39–41]:

■ Muscular rigidity and weakness from immobility
■ Reduced, impaired circulation
■ Constipation, faecal impaction
■ Incontinence
■ Pressure sores
■ Bone demineralization, reduces bone density
■ Reduced metabolic rate
■ Electrolyte losses
■ Death due to strangulation or impaired respiratory function
■ Loss of dignity
■ Loss of sense of well-being

Restraint and falls

Research shows that the risk of falls is constant regardless of policy for or against restraint[39].

Falls are often related to issues of polypharmacy (the adverse effect of taking a number of medications); physical deconditioning, such as loss of muscular strength, balance and range of movement; and trip and slip hazards. So prevention of falls is based on risk management. That is, identifying risks for each person and implementing plans to manage those risks, particularly the environment, e.g. trip hazards, shoes, lighting[39].

Falls are most common:

■ Between noon and midnight
■ Inside person's room
■ Whilst performing activities of daily living: transferring from bed to chair or toilet

Authorising restraint

Depends on country legislative and regulatory requirements, but principally must be from the person being restrained or a person or entity with legal authority.

Continence guidelines

Care staff often have to attend the person with dementia to assist with continence management or address the consequence of incontinence.

Continence care involves the most personal and intrusive care of all activities of daily living and therefore is singled out for specific attention within this book.

Continence

Definition: refers to the ability to voluntarily pass urine or faeces in a socially acceptable place[42–44].

A person is considered to be continent if they:

■ Identify the need to urinate or defecate
■ Spot the toilet
■ Arrive in time to adjust clothing
■ Pass urine or faeces

Urinary continence [42–43, 45]

It is important to understand some basic aspects of normal bladder function to understand incontinence.

- Average volume of urine produced in 24 hours is approximately 1.5 litres.
- Environmental temperature affects urine production, with more urine produced in cold weather.
- Sensation to urinate usually commences when the bladder contains about 200ml of urine (maximum bladder capacity of 400–600ml).
- An average person will urinate 4–6 times daily, though it can be normal to urinate more often.
- Nocturia, urinating at night, is often related to the body's inability to concentrate urine at night. In adults, 25% of urine output is produced at night, which can easily be stored in a healthy bladder. Older people often have to get up twice at night because the kidneys do not effectively concentrate urine at night[44].
- Ageing can lead to a shortening of the period between the sensation to urinate and urinating.
- The kidneys of a person aged 60 years are approximately half as efficient as a person aged 30 years[46].

Incontinence in dementia

Definition: involuntary passing of urine or faeces[42–43].

Contributing factors to incontinence [42–44, 47]

- Cognitive changes, e.g. dementia.
- Physical changes, e.g. reduced mobility or dexterity.
- Sensory changes, e.g. reduced visual acuity and altered spatial perception.
- People with dementia have higher levels of bladder instability.
- Delayed recognition of the period between the initial sensation of needing to pass urine or defecate and the urgent need to urinate or defecate.
- An unfamiliar environment. Orientating to a new environment requires use of short term memory. In a person with dementia this is diminished.
- Patterning a person with dementia to and from the toilet can improve orientation and continence.
- Scheduled toileting in early dementia can lead to contradictory stimuli. For example, routinely toileting a person when there is no urge to urinate may lead to a loss of the concept of the purpose of the toilet. Sitting on a chair with no underwear on may also be taken as a signal to pass urine.
- Stimuli for toileting. Some stimuli may be unfamiliar and therefore inhibit urination or defecation, e.g. sitting on a shower chair or commode.
- Social appropriateness of continence may diminish in a person with moderate to severe dementia, leading to urination or defecation anywhere, possibly including faecal smearing.
- Cognitive and behavioural regression can lead to defensive states, such as bed wetting.
- Ageing can affect the thirst mechanism, so dehydrated older people may not feel thirsty.
- Restricted mobility, including restraint.
- The bladder stretch receptors can also be less efficient in older people. These receptors give the sensation of needing to pass urine and in a healthy adult bladder this occurs when the bladder is about 80–90% full. In the older person there is less warning of the need to urinate and with the loss of elasticity of the bladder the older person can find it more difficult to hold on[46].

Continence assessment [42-45, 48-49]

It is important that a thorough continence assessment is undertaken because research shows that when older people residing in care homes are properly assessed and treated, urinary incontinence can be corrected in 30% of residents and appropriately managed in the remaining population[48]. Assessment minimally incorporates:

■ Person's history of continence
■ Medical history and examination
■ Urine tests
■ Continence charting
■ Aperient charting

Assessments are usually conducted by a registered nurse or a continence nurse adviser with the involvement of members of the multidisciplinary team, such as the general practitioner, physiotherapist and occupational therapist.

Assessment of the person [44-45]

The following factors need to be considered as part of continence assessment. Does the person have?

■ Constipation, faecal impaction or diarrhoea
■ Depression, delirium and/or dementia
■ Diabetes, e.g. polyuria
■ Medication that may cause constipation, diarrhoea or urinary retention
■ Mobility or dexterity issues
■ Urinary tract infection susceptibility
■ Medical history, including surgery

If the person does have incontinence, identify:

■ The normal urination pattern of the person when continent.
■ Periods and location of incontinence when it occurs.
■ Response of care staff in addressing incontinence needs.
■ Aperient regime if incontinent of faeces.

If the person has constipation, consider the following:

■ Faecal bulk can place pressure on the urethra causing outflow obstruction.
■ Faecal bulk can place pressure on the bladder causing urgency and urge incontinence.
■ Faecal bulk can stretch the pelvic floor or distort the angle of the bladder neck causing stress incontinence.
■ Constipation can increase or accentuate confusion.
■ Chronic constipation can lead to impaction, involving continuous overflow of mucus and watery diarrhoea.
■ Adequacy of daily fluid intake.
■ Aperients ordered.

As a first step, where an older person is experiencing incontinence a referral should be made to the registered nurse or continence nurse advisor.

Incontinence can be a symptom of an unsympathetic or challenging environment that prevents the person from toileting. It is also important to consider the following points.

General considerations[48]

- Removing obstacles, e.g. a step into or out of the bathroom.
- Proximity, e.g. shorten the distance from general locality to toilet.
- Mobility aids, e.g. that facilitate turning in bathroom.

Bedroom[42]

- Reduced freedom of movement if safety rails are raised on the bed.
- Low chairs and chairs without arms can hinder mobility.
- Table in front of a chair can hinder mobility.
- Bed too high can hinder mobility.
- Furniture can create obstacles.
- A cold floor or trip hazards can hinder mobility.
- Place the commode adjacent to the bed within easy reach.
- Ensure adequacy of lighting.

Bathroom[42]

- Door signage adequate to differentiate it from other doors.
- Comfortable bathroom temperature.
- Ease of toilet flush.
- Appropriate height of toilet seat, e.g. need for a toilet seat raiser?
- Appropriate lighting level and location of switches for easy reach.
- White toilet on white floor creates lack of contrast so toilet may not be visible.
- Appropriate hand rails for support.
- Adequate manoeuvring space for walking frame or wheelchair.

Temporal routine (care staff activities)[42]

- Vary care staff levels to take account of toileting needs.
- Slow care staff response to request for toileting may lead to incontinence.
- Routine toileting times inconsistent with the person's needs may lead to incontinence.

Clothing[42, 49]

- Preference for clothing that does not require significant fine-motor skills, e.g. velcro or zips, rather than buttons or belts.
- Avoid using difficult-to-manage incontinence pads and pants.
- Avoid using layers of clothing that interfere with access.

Medications[42–43, 47, 49]

Commonly prescribed medications for older persons can disturb bladder function, particularly where polypharmacy is evident, that is, where multiple medications are prescribed.

Careful consideration of the effect of the following is essential:

- Alcohol has a profound sedative effect and also acts as a diuretic. Both these effects may contribute to development of incontinence in vulnerable individuals.
- Caffeine in tea, coffee and cola can irritate the bladder.
- Anticholinergics, such as some antidepressants and phenothiazines, can cause urinary retention leading to overflow incontinence.
- Beta-blockers, prescribed for cardiac conditions such as hypertension, can cause urinary retention leading to overflow incontinence.
- Diuretics, commonly used in the treatment of hypertension, increase urine production and the frequency of voiding.

- Psychotropic medication such as antipsychotics and benzodiazepines can sedate a person, leading to a lack of recognition of the need to urinate. Some of these medications reduce bladder sphincter tone.
- Inappropriate use of aperients can cause incontinence of faeces.

Mobility Issues[42–43]

- Physical limitations arising from acute or chronic health changes can increase the propensity to incontinence. For example, sudden illness or accident, or arthritis and Parkinson's disease.
- Common foot complaints can also increase the propensity to incontinence as they affect balance and comfort, e.g. bunions and corns on the feet.
- Sensory changes, such as macular degeneration, or impaired visual acuity due to dementia, may cause incontinence if the person cannot find or see the toilet.

Continence strategies[47, 49]

Individualised toileting regimens
These are based on anticipated toileting requirements. This involves toileting in advance, that is, toileting thirty minutes prior to anticipated incontinence, based on the person's continence history and assessment. This regimen focuses on the individual's anticipated needs rather then set times.

Scheduled toileting
Scheduled toileting involves toileting at set times, e.g. two hourly. However, this approach can cause incontinence where a person has a normal bladder function.

Bladder retraining
Bladder retraining addresses issues such as frequency and urgency to restore normal bladder function. For bladder retraining consult a continence adviser.

Medical and surgical management
Consideration can be given to medical and surgical intervention. This intervention should be based on a medical history and examination and the holistic impact on the person.

Incontinence strategies

- Pads
  - Are they the correct size for the person?
  - Are they changed regularly?
  - Do they fit comfortably?
- Is there regular hygiene care?
- Is the bowel chart up to date?
- Are aperients reviewed regularly?
- Are regular skin integrity checks made?

Refer to Chapter 4 (the Interaction) for specific techniques related to toileting.

References

1. Trombly, C.A. (1989)
   Occupational Therapy for Physical Dysfunction. Baltimore, William & Wilkins.
2. Ripich, D.N., Petrill, S.A., Whitehouse, P.J. & Ziol, E.W. (1995)
   Gender differences in language of AD patients: a longitudinal study. *Neurology*, 4 (52), 299–302.
3. Buckwalter, J.G., Rizzo, A.A., McCleary, R., Shankle, R., Dick, M. & Henderson, V.W. (1996)
   Gender comparisons of cognitive performances among vascular dementia, Alzheimer disease, and older adults without dementia. *Archive of Neurology*, 53 (5), 436–439.
4. Ott, B.R., Tate, C.A., Gordon, N.M. & Heindel, W.C. (1996)
   Gender differences in the behavioural manifestations of Alzheimer's disease. *Journal of the American Geriatric Society*, 445, 583–587.
5. Ott, B.R., Lapane, K.L. & Gambassi, G. (2000)
   Gender differences in the treatment of behaviour problems in Alzheimer's disease. SAGE Study Group. Systemic Assessment of Geriatric drug use via Epidemiology. *Neurology*, 54 (2), 427–432.
6. Lyketsos, C.G., Steele, C. & Galik, E. (1999)
   Physical aggression in dementia patients and its relationship to depression. *American Journal of Psychiatry*, 156 (1), 66–71.
7. Samuels, R. & Goff, M. (eds) (1998)
   Best Practice Guidelines for the Management of Behavioural Disturbances in Residential Aged Care Facilities. Melbourne, The Royal Australian College of General Practitioners.
8. Burgener, S.C., Bakas, T., Murray, C., Dunahee, J. & Tossey, S. (1999)
   Effective caregiving approaches for patients with Alzheimer's disease. *Geriatric Nursing*, 19 (3), 121–126.
9. Matthews, E.A., Farrell, G.A. & Blackmore, A.M. (1996)
   Effects of an environmental manipulation emphasising client-centred care on agitation and sleep in dementia sufferers in a nursing home. *Journal of Advanced Nursing*, 24 (3), 493–497.
10. Leverett, M. (1991)
    Approaches to problem behaviours in dementia. In: *The Mentally Impaired Elderly: Strategies and Interventions to Maintain Function*. (ed. E.D. Taira) pp. 93–105. New York, The Haworth Press.
11. Palmer, C.V., Adams, S.W. & Bourgeois, M. (1999)
    Reduction in caregiver-identified problem behaviours in patients with Alzheimer disease post-hearing-aid fitting. *Journal of Speech and Hearing Research,* 42 (2), 312–328.
12. Eccles, M., Clarke, J., Livingstone, M., Freemantle, N. & Mason, J. (1998) (Sept)
    North of England evidence-based guidelines development project: guideline for the primary care management of dementia. *British Medical Journal*, 317 (7161), 802–806.
13. Espino, D.V., Jules-Bradley, A.C.A., Johnston, C.L. & Mouton, C.P. (1998) (March)
    Diagnostic approach to the confused elderly patient. *American Family Physician*, 57 (6), 1358–1359.
14. Zal, M. (1999)
    Agitation in the Elderly. *Psychiatric Times*, 16 (1) www.psychiatrictimes.com/p990153.html.
15. Harvey, P.D., Leff, J., Trieman, N., Anderson, J. & Davidson, M. (1997)
    Cognitive impairment in geriatric chronic schizophrenic patients: a crossnational study in New York and London. *Journal of Geriatric Psychiatry*, 12, 1001–1007.
16. Bains, J., Birks, J.S. & Denning, T.R. (2003)
    Antidepressants for treating depression in dementia. (Cochrane Review) *The Cochrane Library*, Issue 3, Oxford, Update Software.
17. Brodaty, H., Draper, B., Saab, D., *et al.* (2001)
    Psychosis, depression and behavioural disturbances in Sydney nursing home residents: prevalence and predictors. *International Journal of Geriatric Psychiatry*, 16, 504–512.
18. Wilson, K., Mottram, P., Sivanranthan, A. & Nightingale, A. (2003)
    Antidepressants versus placebo for the depressed elderly? Issue 3, *The Cochrane Library*, Oxford, Update Issue.
19. Reynolds, C. (1996)
    Making the diagnosis and using SSRIs in the older patient. *Geriatrics*, 51, 28–34.
20. Lanctot, K., Best, T., Mittman, N. & Liu, B. (1998)
    Efficacy and safety of neuroleptics in behavioural disorders associated with dementia. *Journal of Clinical Psychiatry*, 59 (10), 550–561.
21. Brodaty, H., Ames, D., Snowdon, J., *et al.* (2003)
    A randomised placebo-controlled trial of risperidone for the treatment of aggression, agitation and psychosis of dementia. *Journal of Clinical Psychiatry*, 64, 134–143.
22. Draper, B., Snowdon, J., Meares, S., *et al.* (2000)
    Case-controlled study of nursing home residents referred for treatment of vocally disruptive behaviour. *International Psychogeriatrics*, 12 (3), 333–344.

23. Jeste, D.V., Rockwell, E., Harris, M.J., Lohr, J.B. & Lacro, J. (1999)
Conventional versus newer antipsychotics in elderly patients. *American Journal of Geriatric Psychiatry*, 7 (1), 70–76.

24. Kirby, M., Denihan, A., Bruce, I., Radic, A., Coakley, D. & Lawlor, B. (1999)
Benzodiazipine use among elderly in the community. *International Journal of Geriatric Psychiatry*, 14, 280–284.

25. Devanand, D.P., Jacobs, D.M. & Tang, M.X. (1997)
The course of psychopathology in mild to moderate Alzheimer's disease. *Archives General Psychiatry*, 54, 257–263.

26. Grealy, J. & Cody, S. (2000)
An investigation into the prevalence of resistance to care as a cause of staff injury in residential care facilities in South Australia. www.workcover.com.

27. Miller, M.F. (1997)
Physically aggressive resident behaviour during hygienic care. *Journal of Gerontological Nursing*, 23 (5), 24–39, 53–59.

28. White, M., Merrie, J. & Richie, M.F. (1996)
Vocally disruptive behaviour. *Journal of Gerontological Nursing*, 22 (11), 23–29.

29. Kovach, C. & Meyer-Arnold, E. (1997) (May)
Preventing agitated behaviours during bath time. *Geriatric Nursing*, 18 (3), 112–114.

30. Gloth, F.M. (2001)
Pain management in older adults: prevention and treatment. *Journal of the American Geriatrics Society*, 49 (2), 188–189.

31. Monti, D.A. & Kunkel, E.J. (1998)
Management of chronic pain among elderly patients. *Psychiatric Services*, 49 (12), 1537–1539.

32. Gagliese, L. & Melzack, R. (1997)
Chronic pain in elderly people. *Pain,* 70 (1), 3–14.

33. Paris, M. & McLeod, A. (eds) (1999)
Consider the Options: End Stage Clinical Care for Chronic Degenerative Disorders. Adelaide, Hyde Park Press.

34. Feldt, K.S. (2000)
Improving assessment and treatment of pain in cognitively impaired nursing home residents. *Annals of Long Term Care. Clinical Care and Ageing*, 8 (9), 36–42.

35. Huffman, J.C. & Kunik, M.E. (2000)
Assessment and understanding of pain in patients with dementia. *Gerontologist*, 40 (5), 574–581.

36. Streim, J.E., Oslin, D.W., Katz, I.R., *et al.* (2000)
Drug treatment of depression in frail elderly nursing home residents. *American Journal of Geriatric Psychiatry*, 8 (2), 150–159.

37. Hantikainen, V. & Kappeli, S. (2000)
Using restraint with nursing home residents: a qualitative study of nursing staff perceptions and decision making. *Journal of Advanced Nursing*, 32 (5), 1196–1205.

38. Advocare Inc. (2004)
Position Statement on the Use of Restraints in Aged Care Facilities in Western Australia. Perth, Advocare Inc.

39. Dunn, K. (2001)
The effect of physical restraints on falls in older adults who are institutionalised. *Journal of Gerontological Nursing*, 27 (10), 40–48.

40. Karlsson, S., Bucht, G., Rasmussen, B.H. & Sandman, P.O. (2000)
Restraint use in elder care: decision making among registered nurses. *Journal of Clinical Nursing*, 9, 842–850.

41. Hantikainen, V. (2001)
Nursing staff perceptions of the behaviour of older nursing home residents and decision making on restraint use: a qualitative and interpretative study. *Journal of Clinical Nursing*, 10, 246–256.

42. Hunt, S. (ed.) (1993)
Promoting Continence in the Nursing Home: A Resource for Nurses Working in Aged Care. Victoria, Continence Foundation of Australia, Deakin University Publishing Unit.

43. Resthaven Inc. (1996)
Quality Continence Management: A Resource for Carers. Norwood, South Australia, Queen's Court Press.

44. Roe, B. (1994)
Clinical Nursing Practice. The Promotion and Management of Continence. London, Prentice Hall International (UK) Limited.

45. Moody, M (1990)
Incontinence. Patient Problems and Nursing Care. Oxford, Heinemann Nursing.

46. Nazarko, L. (2004)
     Managing continence and minimising complication. *Nursing Residential Care*, 6 (4) 160–166.
47. Norton, C. (ed.) (1996)
     Nursing for Continence 2nd edn. Oxford, Beaconsfield Publishers.
48. Newman, D. (2002)
     Managing and Treating Urinary Incontinence. Baltimore, Health Professions Press.
49. Palmer, M.H. (1996)
     Urinary Continence. Assessment and Promotion. Maryland, Aspen Publishers.

2 The Care Staff

- Model of care
- Contextual interaction
- Communication
- Behavioural reporting
- Lifestyle activities
- References

2 The Care Staff

Model of care

This chapter overviews strategies for effective interaction with persons with dementia, because as dementia progresses there is a reduced capacity to interpret interactions, events, the environment, and to express a response that is consistent with the interaction. The model of care used in this book takes into account the person and three other variables that influence it. These are the care staff, the environment and the interaction, which are summarised below and dealt with in greater depth throughout the book.

(1) The person

- The person with dementia is viewed as an individual with inherent worth.
- The dementia care behaviours are a result of unmet needs of the person with dementia.
- There is a partnership between the care staff and the person with dementia, their family and significant others.

(2) The care staff

- The person with dementia is the focus of care in partnership with the family and friends of the person with dementia.
- The care staff have the responsibility and capacity to identify and respond to the needs of the person.
- The care staff are supported by management and others.

(3) The environment

- The environment is designed with sensitivity to the person with dementia, to provide experiences that are both enriching and meaningful.
- The environment promotes orientation, independence and a sense of security.

(4) The interaction

- Interactions promote an opportunity for the person with dementia for self expression, independence and participation.
- Care staff are skilled to undertake interactions with the person with dementia.

Contextual interaction

Contextual interaction means giving context to the interaction. As the person with dementia can be significantly reliant upon care staff to gain an understanding of the interaction being undertaken, care staff must then become skilled communicators.

This section introduces the term **contextual interaction**.

Contextual Interaction (CI): is a holistic, dementia-specific communication process which uses a number of strategies simultaneously so that the person with dementia has multiple cues to orientate as far as possible to the interaction, which may include orientating to time, place, person and event.

Contextual interaction is comprised of two elements:

(1) **Contextual communication (CC):** verbal and non-verbal forms of communication with the person with dementia focused solely on the goal of the interaction, aimed at orientating the person with dementia to the interaction, which may include orientating to time, place, person, and event.

(2) **Contextual tasking (CT):** a process whereby third party props or objects are used by the care staff member to support the goal of the interaction, aimed at orientating the person with dementia to the interaction, which may include orientation to time, place, person and event.

Contextual communication		Contextual tasking
Verbal communication	**Non-verbal communication**	**Third party props**
■ Voice ■ Tone ■ Pitch ■ Volume ■ Words ■ Rate of speech ■ Verbalised sounds other than speech ■ Structure/order of ideas in a sentence ■ Repeating key concepts	■ Eye movement, direction and contact ■ Facial expression and movements ■ Gestures ■ Body posture and orientation ■ Non-verbal sounds, e.g. clapping ■ Physical appearance such as dress and adornment ■ Posture	■ Use of environment: lighting, climate ■ How one is positioned within the environment ■ Decorations ■ Garments and personal items in the environment, e.g. towel, clothing ■ Smell, odours ■ Soft furnishings pictures, mirrors ■ Food ■ ADL item, cutlery, soap, toilet paper

Communication

Communication is generally a two-way process reliant upon both verbal and non-verbal communication techniques.

Non-verbal forms of communication, such as smiling, grimacing and posture are interpreted by others as outward signs of a person's inner emotions and underlying thoughts, and so can be an effective form of communication.

However, in modern times we communicate a lot of the time without seeing the other person, that is, by telephone, mobile telephones, email, letters and public announcements.

Dementia and communication

Persons with dementia:

■ Often have a heightened awareness of non-verbal forms of communication.
■ Often have an increased sensitivity to the emotion of others.
■ Use or become increasingly reliant upon non-verbal communication techniques to communicate, as the skill of language disappears.

However, as the stages of dementia progress thought structures can also change:

■ Verbal and non-verbal communication may not directly reflect what the person with dementia is trying to express.
■ The person with dementia may not know exactly what they want.
■ The verbal communication may or may not match the non-verbal communication being expressed.

Consequently, it is up to the skilled care staff member to use strategies that increase the likelihood for the person with dementia to understand the meaning:

■ Of what is being communicated (contextual communication: using verbal and non-verbal cues).
■ Of what is happening around them (contextual tasking: using third party props/objects).

This enables the person with dementia to formulate a meaningful response to the information being communicated to them.

The use of a single strategy to communicate, such as verbalising only, is a significantly less effective communication strategy in dementia care than using an approach that incorporates contextual communication, aligning verbal and non-verbal forms of communication, supported by contextual tasking, use of third party props. In the illustration below, Rachael is using words only to communicate in the interaction. Molly, the person with dementia, has a reduced capacity to interpret verbal communication and so her response is inconsistent with Rachael's intent. The outcome is confusion and Molly exhibits resistive behaviour.

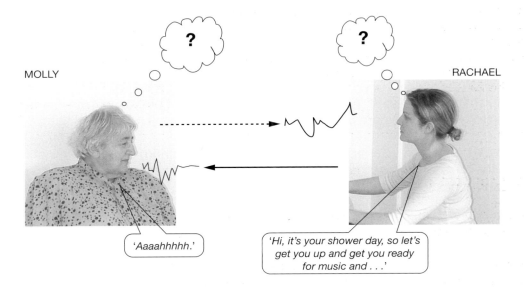

MOLLY

RACHAEL

'Aaaahhhhh.'

'Hi, it's your shower day, so let's get you up and get you ready for music and . . .'

Contextual communication (CC)

Engagement is the first step in contextual communication, and involves:

(1) The care staff getting the person's attention.
(2) Entering the person's world.

(1) The care staff getting the person's attention
Contextual communication requires a visual (sight) and then auditory (hearing) cue to be used first.

(a) **Visual:** position yourself where you can be seen prior to speaking. Establish eye contact.

(b) **Auditory/verbal:** always use the person's name prefixing all sentences and statements. For example, 'Molly, hello, how are you today?' rather than 'Hello, how are you today, Molly?'. Molly may not know you are talking to her if you use her name last.

Refer to the care plan or social history to identify preferred name(s).

(c) **Touch:** use touch, if appropriate, to gain Molly's attention, establish rapport and a sense of friendliness and safety. Initially, only touch neutral places, such as the hand or arm.

Refer to the care plan or social history to identify whether Molly is a tactile person (likes touch).

(d) **Emotion:** establish the emotional relationship with Molly by showing you are happy to see her, and respond to Molly's emotional state. Be careful not to convey negative emotion as Molly may perceive this as your response to her and therefore is more likely to display resistive-to-care behaviour.

(2) Entering the person's world

Generally, the older person with dementia will be occupied prior to the care staff approaching them. Therefore, the person may not immediately be able to change from their activity, understand the request or be able to identify care staff.

Consequently, prior to engaging the person with dementia the care staff member needs to establish, as far as possible:

(a) the predisposition of the person, such as mood and interest in current activity.

(b) the difference between the care staff member's own world and that of the person.

(c) the difference between the current activity of the person and the new activity that the care staff member wants.

(d) decide how they will enter the person's world to begin the interaction.

Remember that the care staff member's relationship with the person with dementia is about the interaction not just the care task.

Care activities are often referred to as tasks, that is, showering, dressing, assisting to eat. However, the term task infers that the care staff member performing the task is active and the other person is passive. This is not true.

The goal of a care activity is the interaction, which may include a task. The interaction is as important to the person being cared for as the outcome of the care activity.

Verbal communication

In contextual communication emphasis is placed on six verbal communication strategies.

(1) Use the person's name first and tell the person who you are.
(2) Identify key words in a care activity and repeat these.
(3) Identify key emotive words in the care activity and repeat these.
(4) Use non-word sounds to convey ideas.
(5) Constant use of appropriate tone, pitch, volume and rate of speech.
(6) Use short sentences and keep instructions simple by discussing one step of the care activity at a time.

These are illustrated below.

(1) Use the person's name first and tell the person who you are.

'Molly, hello. I'm Rachael, your nurse.'

Pleased or happy tone, normal pitch and volume.

(2) Identify key words in a care activity and repeat these.

'Molly, I have your blue *shirt*, it's time to put on your *shirt*.'

Normal conversational tone, normal pitch and volume but emphasise key words.

(3) Identify key emotive words and repeat these.

'Molly, it's time to put on a *warm* shirt and keep *warm*. Molly it's cold today so here is a *warm* shirt. Molly this will make you feel *warm*.'

Normal conversational tone, normal pitch and volume.
Emphasise key emotive words.
(In this context the word 'warm' conveys a sense of comfort.)

(4) Use non-word sounds to convey ideas.

'Molly, it's cold today, *bbbrrrrrrrrr*' and Rachael pretends to shiver.

Non-verbal communication

It is important to note that verbal and non-verbal forms of communication must be aligned for it to be effective and not confusing. What this means, for example, is that if you are smiling when you are telling someone a sad story then the non-verbal signs do not marry with the verbal message and this is confusing to the listener.

Do	Don't
■ Be aware of your own emotional state, are you upset, tired, hurried, hungry? ■ Establish what the person has been doing and respond appropriately. ■ Physically face the person when speaking. ■ Establish eye contact and smile. ■ Give the person an appropriate amount of personal space, then approach. ■ Establish contact by use of touch prior to physical care.	■ Project negative emotion onto the person with dementia as your negative emotion may be interpreted as your feelings about them. ■ Assume the person with dementia can rapidly understand you, understand a sudden new request or intervention if they have been woken only moments before the event. ■ Keep talking when facing away or walking away. ■ Assume that because you have spoken the person knows you are there. ■ Expect the person to immediately allow you to be physically very close. ■ Start care, e.g. transfer the person, as the first form of touch.

An example of contextual communication is illustrated below.

2 The Care Staff

Contextual communication

Verbal communication	Non-verbal communication
(1) Use the person's name first and tell the person who you are.	
'Molly, hello. I'm Rachael, your nurse.'	Rachael starts communication by positioning herself just out of reach giving Molly personal space.
	Rachael makes eye contact, smiles, then approaches and touches Molly's hand/arm making physical but non-threatening contact.
(2) Identify key words in a care activity and repeat these.	
'Molly, I have your blue *shirt*, it's time to put on your *shirt*.'	Rachael makes eye contact with Molly then turns her head and looks at the shirt or touches Molly's upper garment to convey the idea of undressing/dressing.
(3) Identify key emotive words and repeat these.	
'Molly, it's time to put on a *warm* shirt and keep *warm*. Molly it's cold today so here is a *warm* shirt. Molly this will make you feel *warm*.'	Rachael gently strokes Molly's arm to convey warmth.
(4) Use non-word sounds to convey ideas.	
'Molly, it's cold today, *bbbrrrrrrrr*' and the care staff member pretends to shiver.	Rachael pretends to shiver.

Contextual communication is an effective communication approach because it brings together the key concepts and repeats them so that the person with dementia can process simple, orderly, and consistent themes and ideas.

Contextual tasking (CT)

Contextual tasking (CT): involves the use of specific items or props in the environment and the environment itself to orientate the person and prompt a response.

In the scenario given so far the shirt is the third party-prop and is used with verbal and non-verbal communication to reinforce the meaning of the interaction.

For instance, the care staff member shows Molly the shirt, letting Molly touch the shirt or touching Molly with the shirt (on her hand or arm), whilst the care staff member describes getting dressed and staying warm. This is repeated throughout the care process until it is clear that Molly understands the interaction or will accept the care.

When contextual communication and contextual tasking are performed in combination they form contextual interaction.

This is illustrated below.

Verbal communication	Non-verbal communication	Contextual tasking third party props
(1) Use the person's name first. 'Molly, hello. I'm Rachael, your nurse.' Happy tone, normal pitch and volume.	Rachael starts communication by positioning herself just out of reach giving Molly her personal space. Rachael makes eye contact, smiles, then approaches and touches Molly's hand/arm making physical non-threatening contact.	Adjusted lighting and room temperature. Background noise reduced. Prepared clothes and other items needed for care activity.
(2) Identify key words in a care activity and repeat these. 'Molly, I have your blue *shirt*, it's time to put on your *shirt*.' Use normal conversational tone, normal pitch and volume and emphasise key words.	Rachael makes eye contact with Molly, then turns her head and looks at the shirt or touches Molly's upper garment to convey the idea of dressing.	Hold up blue shirt so Molly can see the shirt.
(3) Identify key emotive words and repeat these 'Molly, it's time to put on a *warm* shirt and keep *warm*.' 'Molly it's cold today so here is a *warm* shirt.' 'Molly this will make you feel *warm*.'	Rachael gently rubs Molly's upper arm to convey warmth.	Let Molly touch the shirt. Touch Molly with the shirt, on her hand, arm or cheek of her face, or give Molly an item to hold during the care activity.
(4) Use non-word sounds to convey ideas 'Molly, it's cold today, *bbbrrrrrrrrr*.' Use normal conversational tone, normal pitch and volume and emphasise key emotion).	Rachael pretends to shiver.	

Contextual interaction – bringing it together

A. Preparation

Establish in your mind what needs to be achieved and the order you will take.

Plan the tasks and have items ready.

Adjust the environment if possible or necessary.

If loud music is playing reduce the volume.
Put the bathroom heater on.
Adjust lighting.
Prepare clothing, or other items required.

Prepare yourself emotionally and set your mood. Prepare your focus on the interaction rather than on any concerns.

The emotional content of your speech and behaviour can trigger or lead the person to feel the same, e.g. if impatient, angry, frustrated, these feelings can be taken up by the person and may lead to refusal of care or to leaving the person feeling unwanted or uncared for.

B. Approach

Approach the person diagonally from the front – in their visual range, or if they are seated, squat down to their level.

Physically gain the person's attention prior to or upon talking.

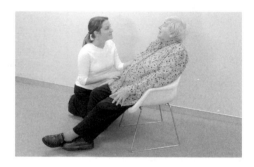

Use the person's preferred name first to prefix communication.

Tell the person who you are, e.g. 'Molly, hello, I'm Rachael your nurse.' And what you are going to do.

Establish non-intrusive physical contact before commencing care.

Speak slowly, clearly and moderate your tone. Present one idea at a time and in logical sequence.

Standing directly in front of the person, face to face, can be misinterpreted as confronting. If the person with dementia is sitting down the care staff member can appear to be towering over the person.

It is recommended that the care staff member approaches the person directly or almost directly in front but once they are about 1–2 metres apart then moves to be diagonally in front of the person with dementia whilst remaining in the person's visual field.

C. Interaction
Establish context to task.

To start the dressing process focus the person's attention on the starting point of the care. For instance, putting the shirt on Molly would involve focusing Molly on her hand.

Avoid asking questions that rely on memory.

Talk about 'now', e.g. don't talk about what happened last time, this can be frustrating for the person if they can't remember last time.

Use non-word sounds to convey ideas.

Allow adequate time for the person to comprehend, respond, request and/or perform activity.

Limit choices, give choices, lead decision making (as necessary).

Tasks need to be broken into simple steps to be successful at each step.

Identify key words in care activity and repeat these.
Hold up blue shirt so Molly can see it.

Use physical cues, such as touching or tapping the older person's hand to focus attention on the hand.

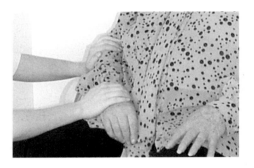

Forearm placement technique.

Rachael cups both hands and places one hand on or near the elbow and the other hand on or near the wrist.

'Molly, it's cold today bbrrrrrr.'

Listen, but also watch the older person's body movements as a sign of understanding.

Choices can be confusing and frustrating – so guide the choice, e.g. 'The blue shirt would be good for church.'

The person may not be able to perform one or more of the steps, so plan to compensate for the inability to perform, e.g. Molly may be able to put on the shirt but cannot do up the buttons.

Checking the response during the interaction

During the interaction it is important that the care staff member continually checks the response of the person with dementia to the interaction.

This checking process helps the care staff member assess how the person will respond; will they be cooperative, uncooperative, passive, or resistive? Listed below are some process checks.

Person	Meaning	General indication
Affect or obvious emotion.	If person is happy or pleased to see you.	Cooperative.
	If the person has a negative mood or affect changes suddenly.	Expect uncooperative.
Response to proposed interaction.	Physically cooperates. Verbally acknowledges.	Cooperative.
	Participating. Assistive.	Cooperative.
	Passive, no specific response.	Cooperative.
	Resists, e.g. pulls away, swears, groans, grimaces.	Resistive.

Contextual interaction: assisting to eat

To further illustrate contextual interaction the example of assisting to eat is presented. These two photographs illustrate the difference between a standard approach and contextual interaction.

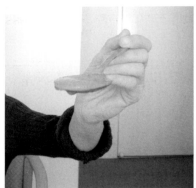

Standard approach to assisted eating: Angela is positioned to the side of the person. In this position the person can only see Angela's hand and spoon.

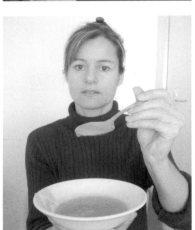

Contextual interaction (assisted eating)
Contextual communication
Verbal communication:

- Angela prefaces each sentence with Molly's name.
- Angela names each item of food on the plate and describes its taste and aroma.
- Conversation focuses on the food and eating.
- Eating is a social activity.

Non-verbal communication:

- Angela smiles, establishes eye contact and sits where Molly can see her.
- Angela initially offers Molly a small taste of the food by placing food on Molly's lips.

Contextual tasking

- In the dining room there are pictures or prints of food.
- On the table there is food, cutlery, placemats, condiments, a serviette.
- There is the pleasant odour of food.
- Lighting is increased.
- Television is turned off.
- Angela shows Molly the food she is about to eat.

2 The Care Staff

The final point to remember when using contextual interaction is to use words that specifically describe an item. For example, use the words 'roast chicken', 'potato', 'carrot', and 'peas', rather than the broad global descriptor of meal or dinner. Otherwise, the person with dementia may not know what is being given to them or what type of food they will be eating.

Global descriptor	Cluster descriptor	Branch descriptor	Specific descriptor
Nutrition	Breakfast	Cereal	Porridge Cornflakes Weetabix
		Drink	Orange juice
Meal	Lunch	Roast	Roast chicken Potato Peas Carrots
		Dessert	Apple pie Ice cream

In this scenario the key emotive words could include:

■ Favourite e.g. 'Your favourite roast chicken.'
■ Delicious e.g. 'The apple pie smells delicious.'
■ Yummy e.g. 'I'm sure that these potatoes taste yummy.'
■ mmm e.g. 'Mmm, the potatoes look great.'

Behavioural reporting

When describing the behaviours of the person with dementia it is important to do the following because it provides clear and objective observational information that assists in determining the cause and triggers of the behaviours and the effectiveness of the interventions.

Record the following:

(1) Date and time.
(2) Care activity and location (interaction).
(3) Describe the person's behaviour using specific behavioural descriptors, e.g. the terms from the RTC risk rating scale.
(4) Duration of behaviour in minutes.
(5) Weight the severity and intensity of the behaviour, e.g. the RTC rating 1, 2, 3 or 4.
(6) Describe the intervention used and its effectiveness.
(7) Initial and designation.

Refer to Appendix 1 for Behavioural Reporting Form.

Lifestyle activities

Lifestyle activities are used to make the person's life more meaningful and should be tailored to meet the person's interests and abilities, and social and cultural needs.

A diversional therapist, lifestyle coordinator or occupational therapist assesses the person's needs and abilities prior to developing a program for them. Listed below are some activities which can be incorporated into the person's therapy programs.

Domestic	Artistic	Outdoor	Reminiscence	Individual	Social
Dust furniture Fold towels Hang out washing Make drinks Wipe off table Fold clothes Prepare morning tea Sort socks Vacuum Iron Bake, biscuits and cakes Polish silverware Make and bake bread	Craft, make a basket, découpage Cut out cards or pictures from magazines Decorate placemats Flower arrangement Paint Read paper	Feed the chooks, dog or cat Plant and care for a garden Rake up leaves Shed activities Sweep the path Take a walk Water plants, garden and lawn Weed the garden	Facials First kiss and hug Hand massage Life review Listen to music Look at photos Manicure Pet visit	Complete an activity board Count things Put a simple puzzle together Sort a deck of cards by suit Sort objects Write a letter	Exercise, ball throwing and catching Invite children to visit Read a letter out loud Laugh Movement, dancing Play quoits Read, poetry Sing hymns, Christmas carols Spelling bee Take a ride Hug a friend

Lifestyle activities is a specialised area; however, there are many activities that a care staff member can incorporate into day-to-day care. Interaction built around meaningful activities can increase the confidence, self-esteem and independence of the person with dementia.

2 The Care Staff

References

For further reading on models of care please see:

1. Alzheimer's Australia (2003)
    Quality dementia care. *Australasian Journal on Ageing*, 22 (4), 203–205.
2. Adams, T. & Manthorpe, J. (2003)
    Dementia Care. London, Arnold Publishers.
3. Andresen, G. (1995)
    Caring for People with Alzheimer's Disease: A Training Manual for Direct Care Providers. Australia, MacLennan & Petty Pty Ltd.
4. Dippel, R. & Hutton, J. (eds) (1991)
    Caring for the Alzheimer Patient. 2nd edn. Buffaho, New York, Prometheus Books.
5. Dowling, J. (1995)
    Keeping Busy . . . A Handbook of Activities for Persons with Dementia. Baltimore, The John Hopkins University Press.
6. Feil, N. (2002)
    Validation Breakthrough 2nd edn. Australia, MacLennan & Petty Pty Ltd.
7. Garratt, S. & Hamilton-Smith, E. (eds) (1995)
    Rethinking Dementia – an Australian Approach. Melbourne, Ausmed Publications.
8. Gruetzner, H. (1988)
    Alzheimer's: A Caregiver's Guide and Source Book. Waco, Texas, John Wiley and Sons Inc.
9. Hellen, C. (1992)
    Alzheimer's Disease: Activity-focused Care. Boston, Andover Medical Publishers.
10. Hoffman, S. & Platt, C. (2000)
    Comforting the Confused: Strategies for Managing Dementia. 2nd edn. New York, Springer Publishing Co.
11. Hunter, S. (ed.) (1997)
    Dementia: Challenges and New Directions. London, Jessica Kingsley Pub.
12. Lubinski, R. (ed.) (1991)
    Dementia and Communication. Philadelphia, B.C. Decker, Inc.

3 The Environment

- Physical and temporal environments
- Environmental requirements
- General considerations
- Bathroom – toilet
- Orientation to own room
- Orientation within own room
- Orientation to dining room
- Orientation to kitchen
- Orientation to lounge room
- Entrances and exits from building
- Internal doors – special care unit, utility and service doors
- Corridors
- Outdoor areas
- Environment to promote interaction
- Environment and walkers
- Environment and confinement
- References

3 The Environment

Physical and temporal environments

The environment is comprised of two related elements:

- Physical
- Temporal

The physical environment refers specifically to the impact building design, materials, colours, climate, lighting and odour have on the person with dementia and others working, living, and or visiting.

The temporal environment refers to the impact people, such as those working and living with, or visiting, have on the person with dementia. An example is cleaning routines and their associated noise.

This section provides an overview of key environmental considerations in the dementia care setting and draws together both the physical and temporal environments.

These guidelines were initially developed in mid-2003 and trialled as part of the project across twelve residential care facilities. The guidelines do not specifically address new environmental design but how to modify existing designs. A Dementia Specific Environmental Audit can be found in Appendix 2. The Audit is based on this section of the book and provides the auditor with a tool to start the process of assessing the environment for its dementia-sensitivity.

Creating a sensitive environment for the person with dementia

The dementia specific environment aims to be sensitive to each person's needs in consideration of their stage of dementia. Therefore, a dementia specific evaluation of the environment must incorporate sensitivity to each person's:

- Memory
- Cognition, including problem-solving skills
- Language
- Activities of daily living
- Coordination skills and physical ability
- Mood and behaviour

The main features of the environment are to:

■ Orientate to the purpose of the area
■ Provide general and focal lighting for tasks
■ Include places for both relaxation and stimulation
■ Occupy the person in a meaningful way
■ Encourage mobility (where appropriate)
■ Promote independence
■ Promote a feeling of security
■ Take account of the person's personality
■ Enhance self-esteem and confidence
■ Be sensitive to each person
■ Facilitate the opportunity for family, visitors and care staff to interact freely with the person

Environmental requirements

These environmental guidelines look at the physical and temporal environments and use the five sub-headings of climate, visual perception, odour/smell, hearing and accessibility to evaluate each area.

Also, under general considerations, special mention is made of noise, lighting and flooring in an attempt to highlight the importance of these three factors in the environment for the person with dementia. For example, persons with dementia need significantly greater lux lighting levels than other adults because their cognitive, sensory and physical changes are often exacerbated by visual degenerative disorders associated with ageing, and so lighting levels in the environment can be used to both signpost objects more clearly or, conversely, obscure them.

For example:

■ The lighting adjacent to a communal toilet may be below the recommended levels, even though the average lux level (level of illumination) for the surrounding area is acceptable and may result in the person being unable to find the toilet door.
■ Lighting levels and light positioning across dining room tables need to take into account shadowing of the food that may occur when the person is seated at the table.
■ The impact of dementia on visual acuity and visual field may raise the consideration for even higher lux levels in certain areas, such as activity and eating areas.

Consultation

The other important aspect of environmental evaluation is consultation. Consultation with:

■ The person with dementia (if possible)
■ The person's guardian or advocate
■ Care staff
■ Manager
■ Clinician
■ Other people who may interact with the person

Consultation with the person with dementia and others helps to ensure that the environment being provided for the person is a meaningful one.

General considerations

Hearing – noise

Loud background noise will frequently have a negative impact on the person with dementia. Noise is most often caused by care staff and others in the environment rather than the physical environment itself.

Lower overall noise level.

■ Lower or remove background music.
■ Turn down loud televisions/radios.
 NB: some people may prefer to have low level of background sound of TV/radio or music rather than silence.
■ Avoid calling out to other care staff and/or visitors.
■ Lubricate squeaky wheels on equipment.
■ Change scheduling of noisy activities when people with dementia are socialising or undertaking specific activities that require concentration, e.g. at mealtimes.
■ Reduce the number of hard surfaces, e.g. carpet communal areas.

Visual perception – lighting

Certain types of lighting can have a negative impact on the person's experience of the environment. A person with dementia generally requires increased lighting levels. However, if that person has macular degeneration, a reduction in lighting may be required. Ongoing assessment of visual acuity will assist in decisions on lighting levels.

Direct glare may be a problem for the person with dementia.

■ Cover light bulbs.
■ For external sunlight causing glare use sheer or translucent curtains.
■ Ensure all windows have a means of filtering or blocking direct sunlight.
■ Install dimmer switches on lights to enable control of lighting levels.

Indirect glare may be a problem for the person with dementia.

■ Use a matt finish or carpet rather than highly polished floors.
■ Cover shiny surfaces or refinish them, e.g. use non-reflective glass on picture frames and on shiny benches.
■ Consider placement of furniture, especially televisions, so sunlight glare from windows is not reflected on them.

3 The Environment

Inappropriate lighting can impact on the person's function and enjoyment.

■ Use daylight adjusted lighting.
■ Install task or focal lighting on tables where the person participates in activities.
■ Use floor lamps at night.
■ Maintain the quality of artificial light by repairing flickering lights or dimming globes, and be aware of the hum associated with fluorescent lighting. Replace as needed.

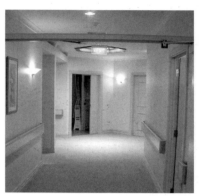

This photograph shows that the skylight focuses light directly onto one area of the floor adjacent to a bedroom that can attract the person/s to enter the bedroom, which may not be desired.

Visual perception – art

The purpose of art is to provide enjoyment and some art can be interacted with.

Attractiveness

▪ Contrast art with the surrounding wall.
▪ Art relevant to the area can assist with orientation, e.g. consider pictures of food in dining areas.
▪ Colours should be clear and well defined, e.g. soft pastel colours can be hard to interpret.

Interaction

Position art to enable the person to interact with it. Art is often hung for an erect adult approximately 170–180cm tall. Many older persons are shorter than this and are stooped.

▪ Art should be positioned to enable the seated person to see and possibly touch the art.
▪ Focal lighting over art can draw attention to the art and therefore occupy the person.
▪ Abstract art may be difficult to interpret and have limited meaning.
▪ Consider art that is age relevant.
▪ Consider installing non-reflective glass over prints.

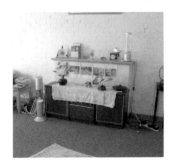

This area could be confusing to the person with dementia because it is cluttered.

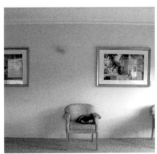

The prints on this wall are hung at a height for an adult standing 170–180cm tall. Notice the glare on the glass in the print on the left, which obscures the picture. Two solitary chairs face away from the prints.

Visual perception – colour

The person with dementia may have difficulties discerning edges in rooms, and where the wall finishes and the floor begins.

■ Use mixed light sources to improve overall lighting levels.
■ Full-spectrum fluorescent and incandescent globes reduce eye fatigue and provide good colour rendering.
■ Incandescent globes provide warmer, cosier atmospheres but are not recommended as a primary light source.
■ Frosted incandescent globes diffuse light and reduce glare.
■ Edges of items are less visible in indirect light.
■ Contrast floor and wall colours.

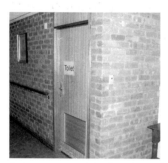

Similar colours and hues of door, wall and floor can reduce orientation to the environment.

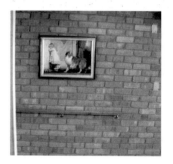

The brown handrail is disguised by the brown wall, making it very difficult for the person with visual impairment to see it. The picture is predominantly brown, with a brown frame, and so is disguised by the brown wall. The picture is hung for a 170–180cm adult person. This is too high for the older person to see it properly.

Visual perception – flooring

Flooring design and type can promote mobility and a sense of safety, whilst inappropriate flooring can negatively impact upon a person's function, enjoyment and mobility.

- A change in flooring material or pattern can appear as an obstacle to some people with visual and/or cognitive impairment.
- Contrasts between floor material and joins, e.g. black lines can appear as unsafe and can interfere with the person's mobility.
- Vivid patterns can be confusing.
- Highly polished surfaces may appear unsafe, e.g. reflected light may appear to the person as water on the floor, thereby interfering with the person's mobility.

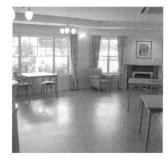

Direct external sunlight and internal lighting can cause glare to be reflected on polished floors. Glare can give the appearance of water on the floor, which can affect mobility.

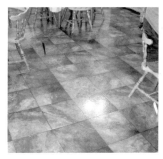

Internal lighting glare from a down light in the dining room gives the appearance of spilled water on the floor.

Bathroom – toilet

The main purpose of the bathroom and toilet is for personal hygiene and these are generally considered private activities. The person with dementia needs to be able to recognise the primary purpose of the bathroom and toilet and therefore the environment should support and reinforce this purpose.

Climate

■ Bath areas need to be warmer than adjacent and public areas. Install heat lamps or radiant heat panels to allow for adjustment of temperature, as these can provide supplemental heat to make the bathroom more comfortable.

Visual perception

■ Install large light switches that contrast with the wall and locate at the entry opposite the swing of the door making it easier for the person to locate and reach the switch.
■ Install sensor lights that activate on approach, and that have a long 'on' period as this prevents the light going off when a person is stationary on the toilet.
■ Heat lamps and bright lights can create glare off shiny white tiles and from the floor. Very bright lighting can make it difficult to see a white toilet seat with a white or grey floor, as, for the person with dementia, it all blurs into one.
■ Include items of visual interest, such as indoor plants, mirrors, colourful towels and colourful privacy curtains.

Odour/smell

■ Ensure bathrooms are fresh and/or fragrant smelling. Indoor plants, soaps and air fresheners can assist with this.

Hearing

■ Reduce noise levels, such as noisy extractor fans, and dampen bathroom echo if it is an issue for the person.
■ For some people soft background music improves the ambience of the bathroom.

Accessibility

■ Consider hand-held shower wands, or adjust height or direction of the showerhead to offer flexibility for the person in washing.
■ Include items of visual interest, with plants, mirrors, towels, privacy curtains and aromas or scents that make the bathroom area attractive to the person.
■ Contrast the colour of the toilet seat with floor, the colour of the hand basin with the surrounding bench, and the shower recess with bathroom floor. This enables the person to distinguish objects in the bathroom.
■ If the bathroom floor is cold, place bathmats or a similar item on the floor so the person does not have to walk barefooted on a cold floor.
■ Install grab rails, non-slip floor and call bell.
■ Install a small shelf in the shower recess, positioned at mid-abdomen level of the person seated on a shower chair. This provides for personal items to be within their reach.
■ Cylindrical tap handles can increase orientation because they may be familiar, but can be more difficult to use than lever taps.
■ Install a mirror at a height that a seated person at the hand basin can see, and increase lighting over this mirror.

■ Consider installing a mirror that can be reversed to a solid finish because mirrors can leave different impressions on the person with dementia. The person may like seeing themself, or they may not recognise themself in the mirror, which can cause distress, or the person may be indifferent to mirrors.

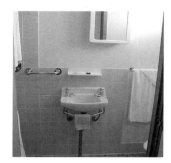

In this bathroom the mirror is positioned too high for the person who is seated to see themselves. It is also not directly parallel with the basin. Note that there is also insufficient shelf space for personal items.

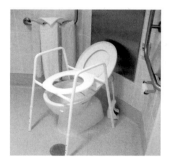

This photograph shows the lack of contrast of colour between the white toilet seat, its base and the grey floor. Use of heat lamps act to further decrease contrast of toilet seat in the bathroom. This lack of contrast makes it very difficult for the person to see the toilet.

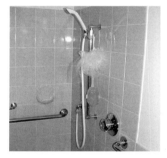

In this shower recess there is no space for personal items and the shower rose and hose is positioned very high up on the wall. Note the cylindrical tap handles.

3 The Environment

Orientation to own room

The main purpose of corridors and passages is to facilitate movement from one place of purpose to another. The corridor and passage may also provide opportunities to interact with others or, if there is seating, act as rest points. Therefore, corridor and passage design leading to rooms needs to assist the person to locate their own room with little or no difficulty.

Climate

▪ Maintain a temperature suitable for the person rather than the care staff or visitor, and adjust climate control over the day. The person may not like to enter a room with a different temperature from the corridor or passage.

Visual perception

▪ Place signs on the section of the door where the person is most likely to see it. If their range of vision is limited this might be quite low, such as 100cm from the floor.

▪ Or place a sign or item that the person recognises or finds interesting in the bedroom, which is clearly visible from the door, to encourage the person to enter the room.

▪ Consider signage that includes both symbols and written words.

▪ It is preferable that written words are in title case rather than capitals, e.g. Elizabeth, as it is easier to read.

▪ Names may need to be the first name or abbreviated first name of the person. For example, Mrs Elizabeth Smith may not remember her name as Mrs Smith. She may only recall her name as Beth.

▪ Large light switches that colour contrast with the wall and are located at the entry opposite the swing of the door and no greater than shoulder height of the person make it within their reach and can be easily located.

Odour/smell

▪ Ensure the room is fresh and/or fragrant smelling.

▪ Consider using their favourite scent or other familiar smells as a cue for the person to identify their own room.

Hearing

▪ Use music that the person finds familiar, so that a person may find their room partly by hearing that particular music.

Accessibility

▪ Contrast the colour of the bedroom door with adjacent doors and walls, as beige walls and beige doors may be difficult for the person to distinguish between.

▪ Personal orientation cues help the person recognise their room and these should be well lit, e.g. pictures, photographs or ornament.

▪ Lever action door handles are generally easier to manipulate than cylindrical door handles.

▪ Avoid marked contrast in colour and pattern between flooring colour from the corridor into the bedroom because the point where a dark colour meets a light colour can appear as a step.

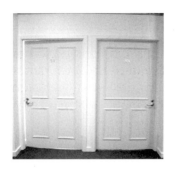

Identical coloured doors with no signposting or distinguishing features can be disorientating to the person.

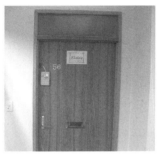

In this photograph the person's name has been placed well above normal visual range.

Orientation within own room

The bedroom has multiple purposes, but primarily acts as a personal space belonging to the person. The bedroom may be used for rest, relaxation, entertainment of visitors and private activities. The person needs to be able to recognise the bedroom as their own and, if shared, that there is a space within the room that belongs to them, and therefore the environment can help reinforce this purpose.

Climate

■ Maintain a temperature suitable for the person rather than the care staff or visitor, and adjust climate control over the day. The person may not remain in a very cold or hot room.

■ Preference for open or closed windows needs to be determined and incorporated in care plans.

Visual perception

■ Place furniture in the room that the person finds familiar and is suited to their physical ability.

■ Personalise the room with their choice of
  ■ quilt cover/blankets
  ■ photographs and prints
  ■ at least one piece of art or photograph on a wall or side cupboard that the person lying on their side in bed can see
  ■ a familiar piece of clothing on the bed or art object on the bed head to show that the bed belongs to that person

■ Place a large light switch that colour contrasts with the wall so that it is located at the entry opposite the swing of the door. Switch placement should not be higher than the shoulder height of the person.

■ Consider the need to adjust curtains to prevent sunlight glare during the day.

■ Ensure access to other light switches for focal lighting needs, such as a bed lamp or chair lamp.

Odour/smell

■ Keep the bedroom fresh and/or fragrant smelling. Open windows help freshen a room.

■ Consider using their favourite scent or familiar smells as cues for the person to identify their own room.

Hearing

■ Play music in the room that the person finds familiar as this helps increase their sense of enjoyment of being in their room.

■ Play music that is calming and promotes rest during rest periods, e.g. classical music.

Accessibility

■ Contrast the colour of the bedroom door with adjacent doors and walls, as beige walls and beige doors may be difficult to distinguish between.

■ Lever action door handles are generally easier to manipulate than cylindrical door handles.

■ Avoid marked contrast in colour and pattern between flooring colour from the corridor into the bedroom because the point where a dark colour meets a light colour can appear as a step.

- Non-slip matting for non-carpeted areas can improve stability and it also reduces the cold feeling of floor on bare feet.
- Reduce clutter to improve access to all areas of the room.
- Provide accessible storage, such as a wardrobe clearly signposted, and items on hangers at the height of the person so they can reach their clothes. For example, if the rack is 180cm high and the person is 150cm tall, lower the rack.
- Place commonly used items within reach, including shoes in the cupboard rather than below knee level or above shoulder height.
- Most falls occur between midday and midnight and often in the person's own bedroom. Consider making a clear passage from the bed to the toilet or commode and increase lighting in the bathroom, perhaps installing a sensor light with a long 'on' period.

Orientation to dining room

The main purpose of the dining room is for eating meals, which may include socialising. Some dining rooms are also used for other purposes, such as an activity area or as a combined dining-lounge room. The person needs to be able to recognise the primary purpose of the dining area.

Climate

■ Maintain a temperature suitable for the person rather than the care staff or visitor, and adjust climate control over the day. The person may not want to stay in the dining area if there are cool drafts or the room temperature is too warm or too cold.

Visual perception

■ Ensure that the dining area has visual cues that reinforce the purpose of the area as one of eating meals and socialising, e.g. condiments on the table.
■ Artwork of food in the environment can help reinforce the purpose of the area and facilitates items of interest for care staff to talk to the person about. Mealtimes can then be used as a process of orientating the person and stimulating the person's appetite.
■ Placemats can help define the person's eating area but be aware that round placemats can be mistaken for plates.
■ Increased lighting over tables at mealtimes assists the person in seeing the food and other items on the table.

Odour/smell

■ Food aromas help stimulate appetite.
■ To increase appetite and orientation, the care staff member can repeat key words that help the person understand what type of food they are about to eat. For example, 'Molly, your roast chicken looks good and smells good too. Roast chicken is your favourite meal.'

Hearing

■ Particularly for the visually impaired person, encourage care staff to talk about the menu to the person before they commence eating. Describe the food on their plate and how it might taste to help stimulate appetite.
■ Consider using background music that the person finds familiar and has a slow rhythm to enhance the dining experience.
■ Try to avoid calling out or speaking loudly as it may distract the person from eating.

Accessibility

■ It helps to serve food that contrasts with the colour of the plate. That is, try to avoid placing white food in white bowls or plates. The plate should also contrast with the colour of the placemat, and placemat with the table. This helps the person identify their food, their plate and eating area on the table.
■ Try to avoid tablecloths and placemats that have flower patterns (flowers are meant to be picked) or busy patterns, which may be confusing.
■ Try not to rush when serving as this may distract the person from eating.
■ Provide tables to seat four people and a maximum of six people and have some tables to seat one or two people that allow the person to choose their seating preference.

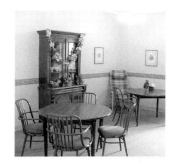

Discrete seating of 4–6 persons promotes opportunity for social-isation, and/or seating for one which provides seating choice.

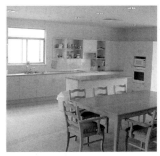

Note the proximity of the dining area to the kitchen. This helps reinforce the purpose of the dining room and facilitates orientation to place.

3 The Environment

Orientation to kitchen

The main purpose of the kitchen is the preparation of meals, followed by socialising and therapy programs for the person. The person needs to be able to recognise the primary purpose of the kitchen.

Climate

■ As the temperature may be higher in the kitchen than adjacent areas it may be necessary to undertake some activities nearby.

Visual perception

■ Ensure that the kitchen area has visual cues that reinforce the purpose of the area as one of food preparation and cleaning up.
■ Increased lighting over benches and sinks assists the person in seeing the food and other items on the bench and in the sink.
■ Preferably have crockery and cooking dishes that contrast with the bench so that the person can clearly see them.
■ When undertaking any cooking activity, reduce clutter, e.g. remove items not in use to help focus the person on the immediate activity.

Odour/smell

■ Food and cooking aromas help stimulate appetite.
■ Talk about the food aromas to increase appetite and orientation.

Hearing

■ Describe the activity by providing verbal and physical prompts of the steps in the cooking process.
■ Reduce or turn off background noise as this can distract the person from the program.

Accessibility

■ Safety is a key concern in the kitchen so undertake a risk assessment and implement a risk management program for all aspects of the kitchen.
  Consider safety features such as:
    ■ hot water temperature control valve
    ■ electrical and gas isolation of all appliances
    ■ coded microwave ovens to prevent use when unsupervised
    ■ an over-ride switch to control dishwasher
    ■ isolation of poisons
    ■ increased lighting over task areas
    ■ only using crockery that has a safety rating
    ■ securing sharp items until supervised
    ■ an audible alarm on the refrigerator door to indicate when it has been left open longer than 90 seconds
■ Have available small portions of food and fluid for the person to snack on.
■ Leave familiar items in the kitchen, e.g. tea towels, dish rack, safe cooking utensils, e.g. wooden spoons, as these help to orientate the person to place.

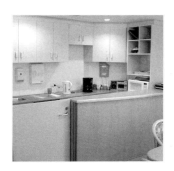

This kitchen is located in the middle of a dining room. It has a very high level of lighting, and care staff stand here at times. The lighting and the presence of staff attract the person to enter the kitchen. However, a locked barn door to the kitchen can be frustrating for the person.

Orientation to lounge room

The main purpose of the lounge room is for socialising, which can involve passive activities, such as sitting quietly, reading, watching television and listening to music, or it may involve participative activities, such as talking and therapy programs. Some lounge rooms are also used for other purposes, such as activity areas or as a combined dining-lounge room. The person needs to be able to recognise the primary purpose of the lounge area and the environment can help reinforce this purpose.

Climate

■ Maintain a temperature suitable for the person rather than the care staff or visitor, and adjust climate control over the day. The person may not want to stay in a lounge room if there are cool drafts or the room temperature is too warm or too cold.

Visual perception

■ Artwork within the environment, of portraits or landscapes, flowers or people gathered together, reinforces the purpose of the area and provides items of interest for care staff to talk to the person about.
■ Engaging the person in social activities in the room assists in orientation.
■ Position some non-hazardous art objects next to lounges at the seated person's head height and if possible within their reach. This increases the opportunity for the person to interact with the art and the environment.
■ Increase lighting over chairs and tables where activities are carried out.

Odour/smell

■ Aromatherapy and essential oils can be used to stimulate or relax.
■ Fresh air can improve the ambience of the lounge room.

Hearing

■ Care staff can help orientate the person by talking about the comfort of the room, the view from the window, the type of art on the walls and/or the activities underway in the room.
■ Background music may help maintain a settled and interesting environment. Television noise can have mixed effects and needs to be carefully monitored.
■ Try to avoid calling out or speaking loudly if the ambience of the room is a peaceful one.

Accessibility

■ Have small individual activities available for the person who is looking for something to do.
■ Consider arranging furniture to encourage the person to sit down and rest. Two chairs angled together with a coffee table in between can encourage socialisation, and place items of interest on the coffee table and increase focal lighting in that area.
■ Try to avoid positioning furniture, such as a single chair or chairs, with their back to the wall, as this does not allow the person to see or interact with art objects on the wall behind.
■ Use of contrasting colours between doorways, door handles, doors, wall edges and light switches assist the person to identify door entries and exits.
■ Consider contrasting the furniture to increase the interest in the lounge room.
■ It is preferable that flooring colour and pattern in the lounge room be consistent.

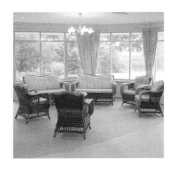

This lounge room is well positioned, brightly lit and easily accessible to the person.

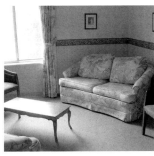

In this photograph the arrangement of the furniture in a circle and the contrast of sofa and single chairs encourage socialisation, as more than two people can sit together. Note that there are no objects or items of interest to occupy a single person seated alone.

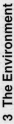

3 The Environment

Entrances and exits from building

The main purpose of the entrance and exit door is to enter or leave the building. It is important to determine which door(s) the person should have access to and how to facilitate this access. The person needs to be able to recognise the primary purpose of the exit door and therefore the environment can be used to reinforce this purpose.

Climate

■ If seating is situated near egresses, cool drafts may stop the person sitting and resting. Place egress seating clear of the door swing and away from cool drafts.

■ Sudden changes in temperature when moving from inside to outside can diminish the positive experience for the person. Consider installing an air lock between internal and external doors which allows for adjustment in temperature.

Visual perception

To reduce accessibility:

■ Lower lighting at the door and adjacent area.

■ Install a solid door similar to internal doors to disguise it.

■ Paint the exit door the same colour and finish as the surrounding walls.

To increase accessibility:

■ Contrast colour and style of the door from the walls and flooring. Perhaps consider having a glass insert in the door so the older person can see out.

■ Increase lighting at the entrance and exit doors during the day.

■ Use specific exits consistently throughout the day and avoid using exits that the person should not use.

■ Provide a comfortable seating area for the person to adjust to lighting levels before moving outside.

■ Leave entrance and exit doors open during the day, in consideration of there being secure areas beyond in which the person can remain safe.

Odour/smell

To reduce accessibility:

■ Prevent outside odours from entering the building.

To increase accessibility:

■ Fresh air can improve the ambience of the environment.

■ Scented plants or shrubs adjacent to the door or in gardens on the other side of the door act as attractions.

Hearing

To reduce accessibility:

■ Care staff and others should avoid standing and talking at the door as this can attract people to the door.

■ Announcing out loud or calling out that you are leaving the building, such as 'I'm going home now,' might be interpreted by the person as being their time to leave also.

To increase accessibility:

■ Standing and talking at the door and describing the outside environment to the person may encourage them to walk outside.

■ Having a seating area on the external side of the door may attract the person to walk through the door and sit outside.

Accessibility

To reduce accessibility:

- Remove the door handle and replace with key lock or a coded pad.
- Remove the door sign and place above the door out of visual range of the person.
- Consider removing the part of the door architrave that sits proud of the wall and is visible in the corridor.
- Paint the colour of the door the same colour as the surrounding walls to disguise it.

To increase accessibility:

- Flooring between internal and external areas should be a similar colour and there should be no step/s or trip hazard/s.
- Arrange comfortable furniture to encourage the person to sit either inside or outside.
- Consider automatic doors or doors with lever door handles that can be turned easily.

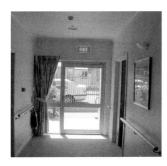

Sunlight entering the building through external doors can act to attract the person to it.

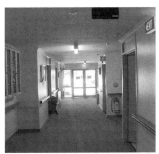

In this photograph the sunlight streaming through the front glass doors of the building highlights one end of the corridor, giving it a tunnel-like effect which will subsequently attract the person to walk towards the lit end.

3 The Environment

Internal doors – special care unit, utility and service doors

The main purpose of these doors is for care staff and others to enter or leave, and they are generally off limits to the person with dementia for safety reasons. It is important, then, to determine which door(s) the person with dementia cannot have access to. The following suggestions show how to reduce accessibility to these specific doors within a building.

Climate

■ Not applicable.

Visual perception

■ Lower lighting at the door and adjacent area.
■ Install a solid door similar in style to other internal doors.
■ Paint the door the same colour and finish as the adjacent walls.
■ Remove the architrave that sits proud of the wall into the corridor.
■ Cover light entering from the other side of the door. For example, if light from a utility room beams into the corridor through a glass panel in the door consider:
    ■ removing or covering the glass panel if safe to do so
    ■ reducing the lighting level in the utility room
    ■ increasing lighting along the length of the corridor so the light entering the corridor is not isolated
    ■ installing a sensor light in the room so light activates upon approach and entry rather than being constant
    ■ covering any sky lights if appropriate
    ■ turning off the light when not in the room

Odour/smell

■ Mask or prevent interesting smells from entering the surrounding areas.

Hearing

■ Care staff and others should try not to stand at the door for long periods as this may attract the person to the door.
■ Try not to call out loudly when you are at the door. For example, 'I'm just popping in here for a minute,' as this might attract the person to follow you inside.

Accessibility

■ Remove door handle and replace with key lock or coded pad.
■ Remove the door sign and place above the door or with small symbol above 180cm height.
■ Remove door architrave that is visible in the corridor.
■ Paint the door the same colour and finish as the adjacent walls.
■ Contrast the flooring between the two areas.
■ Remove furniture or seating placed near the door.

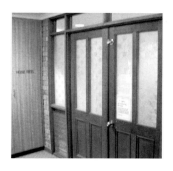

Well lit and interesting doors to special care units (SCUs) tend to attract the person to them.

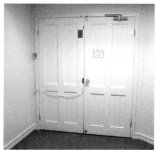

Painting the door the same colour and finish as the adjacent wall acts to disguise the door.

Service doors

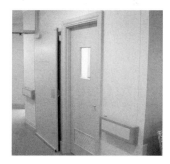

Light streaming out of a utility room window or door into the corridor can attract the person to it.

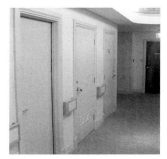

In this photograph the utility door is the same colour as the toilet door. This can be disorientating to the person as they cannot distinguish which door is the toilet door.

3 The Environment

Corridors

The main purpose of corridors/passages is to facilitate movement from one place of purpose to another. The corridor/passage may also provide opportunities to interact with others or, if there is seating, to act as rest points.

Climate

■ Cool drafts from open doors, air conditioning ducts and windows may make being in corridors uncomfortable. Regularly check to ensure the temperature is comfortable for the person.
■ Maintain a temperature similar to other communal areas.

Visual perception

■ Provide lighting of even distribution along the corridor, to avoid shadowing caused by direct down lights, or bright external light streaming across a section of the corridor.
■ Relevant doors along the corridor can be painted a contrasting colour. For example, the colour of the toilet door can be a brighter colour than the corridor walls to allow for easy identification.

Odour/smell

■ Keep utility and service doors along the corridor closed at all times to prevent odours from entering the corridor and attracting the person.

Hearing

■ Care staff and others can encourage mobility of the person in the corridor by walking with them and discussing art objects and/or prints on the walls, to increase the enjoyment of exercising and/or of their environment.

Accessibility

■ Contrast the colour of the corridor walls from the flooring so it is clear where the wall begins.
■ Use contrasting colours in the environment as a way of helping the person find specific doorways, such as the toilet, dining and lounge rooms.
■ Have a consistent coloured floor in the corridor, with no heavy patterns or lines that may be interpreted by the person as steps or hazards.
■ Along the corridor provide rest and activity areas that are clearly visible to the person. For example, arrange comfortable chairs along the corridor to encourage the person to walk the full length of the corridor if possible, and take many rest stops. Place items of interest along the way that are not trip hazards, and increase focal lighting at chairs and on wall artwork at eye level so the pieces can be seen clearly when sitting.
■ Consider using different style door handles and door colours for different rooms.

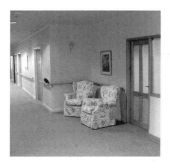

This photograph shows how rest points have been set up along a corridor for the mobile person.
This encourages both mobility and rest stops.

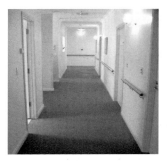

In this photograph note that the handrails are clearly visible and are in a contrasting colour to the wall colour.

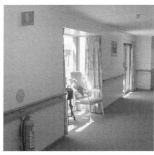

A dark corridor where walls, floor and doors are similar depth of colour and hue can reduce orientation.

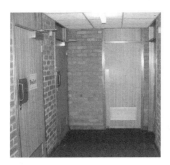

In this photograph note the long corridor with no visible rest points or items of interest on the walls. A high level of light entering the corridor from bedrooms may also attract the person to enter another person's room.

3 The Environment

Outdoor areas

Outdoor areas have a number of purposes, including walking, sitting or recreational and social activities. It is important to determine how the person accesses and leaves the external area and how they orientate themselves to the purpose of the area.

Climate

- Provide covered and exposed walkways for year round access.
- Provide seating in exposed and covered areas for year round access.
- Shelter from wind, drafts and rain should be considered.

Visual perception

- Provide interesting colour-scapes by selecting and grouping colourful plants and flowers.

Odour/smell

- Aromatic gardens can improve the ambience of the environment, using scented plants or shrubs.

Hearing

- Waterscapes can attract and occupy the person, e.g. a fountain, small waterfall or pond.
- Consider establishing a bird aviary.

Accessibility

- Solid, unbroken paths, e.g. concrete with continuous colour, encourages mobility.
- Segment garden into functions, e.g. scented garden, waterscape, colour-scape, for interest.
- Have rest points positioned so a place is in sight at all times when walking on the path(s).
- Paths should end at an entrance to the building rather than a locked gate.
- Obscure the fence with shrubs to reduce the sensation of being fenced in.
- Raised garden beds give access to garden when seated. Consider a structure that allows the person to sit alongside the raised garden bed.
- A vegetable garden can elicit purposeful activity.
- Consider having vegetation that is not poisonous.
- Consider other items of interest, such as a mock bus stop, a garden shed and or an outside workbench.
- A playground can provide a medium for the person to passively and or actively interact with children and their parents.
- A barbecue area and outdoor chairs and tables provide ready access to an outdoor dining area.
- Fruit trees and vegetable gardens provide seasonal fresh fruit and vegetables.
- All areas should be designed for wheelchair access.

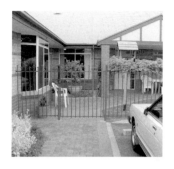 In this photograph the pathway ends at a locked gate, which may give the person a sense of confinement.

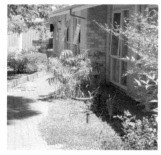 In this photograph it is unclear where the meandering path leads to. Also, note that the ground cover has started covering the path, which may hinder mobilisation.

3 The Environment

Environment to promote interaction

The environment can promote interaction and communication between the person and others. One way this can be done is by arranging furniture to promote the opportunity of social interaction. Seating may be placed for two people, with a table in between, to enable them to have a drink, play a game or glance through magazines. Or seating may be arranged to encourage many people to gather together to share an activity. Having interesting objects on tables or within the environment can also help facilitate conversation.

Environment and walkers

The environment can address the needs of a person who wanders. The environment can be made to directly or indirectly engage the person. This can be done by hanging interactive art objects along the most frequently travelled routes, such as the corridor, and placing comfortable chairs along the corridor to encourage the active person to stop and rest periodically. You might also like to consider scheduling familiar activities for the person that they can enjoy, to break their walking. Also, remember that the environment can provide opportunities to aid nutrition to overactive walkers. Place drinks or snacks in common areas.

Environment and confinement

It is important that the environment maximises freedom of movement and expression for the person with dementia.

- Does the environment promote a positive experience for the person?
- Does the environment give them a sense of comfort and safety?
- Is the environment meaningful to the person?
- Is their independence maximised?
- Is there a secure outside area where the person can come and go as they please?
- Visual sites like a garden, garden furniture and sculpture, such as water fountains or ponds, can increase the enjoyment and interest of being outside.
- Is there sufficient space to walk around with a walking frame or wheelchair?
- Are there rest spots along frequently travelled routes?
- Are there quiet times or rest periods during the day in which calming classical music is played to help reduce agitation in some persons?
- Can the person move easily and freely between unrestricted areas?
- How often is the person encouraged to do activities outside their own room?
- Are supervised outings during the week organised so that the person, if able to, can go?
- Is social interaction between the person and their friends and family members encouraged and supported?

References

1. Alzheimer's Australia (2003)
   Quality Dementia Care Position Paper 2: www.alzheimers.org.au
2. Alzheimer's Australia (2004)
   Dementia Care and the Built Environment: www.alzheimers.org.au
3. Bassi, C.J., Solomon, K. & Young D. (1993)
   Vision in ageing and dementia. *Optometry and Vision Science*, 70 (10), 809–813.
4. Brawley, E.C. (1997)
   Designing for Alzheimer's Disease: Strategies for Creating Better Environments. London, John Wiley and Sons.
5. Calkins, M. (2001)
   Creating Successful Dementia Care Settings Vols 1–4. Baltimore, Health Professions Press.
6. Cohen, U. & Day, K. (1993)
   Contemporary Environments for People with Dementia. Baltimore, The John Hopkins University Press.
7. Cohen-Mansfield, J. & Werner, P. (1998)
   The effects of an enhanced environment on nursing home residents who pace. *The Gerontologist*, 38 (2), 199–208.
8. Cooper, B.A. (1999)
   The utility of functional colour cues, *Scandinavian Journal of Caring Science*, 13, 186–192.
9. Cooper, B.A., Mohide, A. & Gilbert, S. (1989)
   Testing the use of color. *Dimensions*, Sept. 22–26.
10. Cronin-Golomb, A. (1995)
    Vision in Alzheimer's disease. *The Gerontologist*, 35 (3), 370–376.
11. Julian, W. & Verriest, G. (1997)
    Lighting Needs for the Partially Sighted, Vienna CIE Publication 123.
12. Malkin, J. (1992)
    Hospital Interior Architecture, New York, Van Nostrand Reinhold.
13. Marshall, M. (1998)
    Environment: how it helps to see dementia as a disability (ed. S. Benson) *The Journal of Dementia Care*, 6 (1) (Jan.–Feb.), 15–17.
14. Williams, M. (1988)
    The physical environment and patient care, *Annual Review of Nursing Research*, 6, 61–84.

4   The Interaction

- Repositioning in bed
- Transfer from lying to sitting no. 1
- Transfer from lying to sitting no. 2
- Mechanical hoist
- Stand transfer
- Correcting sitting posture
- Wheelchair mobilising
- Continence pad change – standing
- Continence pad change in bed no. 1
- Continence pad change in bed no. 2
- Toileting
- Showering
- Dressing
- Putting shoes on
- Assisting to eat
- Eating
- Sundowning
- Catastrophic reaction
- Wandering
- Hitting – standing
- Hitting – squatting
- Throwing

Please read

These twenty-two interactions have been chosen because they were identified in the project as being of most concern to care staff. The interactions are a guide only. Don't forget to review these procedures to ensure that they fit within your own organisation's policy and practices prior to use.

ADL – activities of daily living
RTC – resistance to care

4 The Interaction

Repositioning in bed

ADL:	**Repositioning in bed**
RTC:	**Grabbing soft items or fixtures**
Technique:	**Loosening grip**
Number of care staff:	**1**

Possible triggers of RTC:

- Seeking a sense of security.
- Misunderstands the care interaction.
- The person does not want to move.

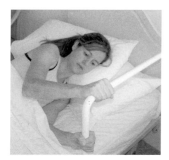

Angela demonstrates grabbing a safety rail whilst in bed.

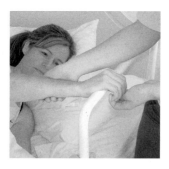

Lifting Angela's fingers from the rail, finger by finger, will lead to tightening of her grip and possible injury to Angela.

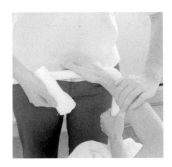

To disengage Angela's grasp Rachael distracts Angela first, then gently strokes Angela's forearm.
Gentle stroking will decrease muscle tension in Angela's arm and hand and lead to her loosening her grip on the rail.

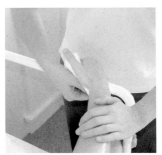

As Angela loosens her grip on the rail Rachael slips a soft item in her hand, e.g. a rolled face flannel.
This technique reduces the chances of Angela grabbing for the safety rail or other items because her hand is occupied.

✓ **Key Learning:** Repositioning in bed		
Contextual communication		**Contextual tasking**
Verbal communication	**Non-verbal communication**	**Third party props**
Distract the person by drawing her attention away from the rail to a photograph or other item nearby.	Gently stroke Angela's forearm using your fingers, a tissue or cotton wool, if available.	Dimmed lighting. Warm room temperature. Quiet environment.
Explain the care activity you are about to undertake, 'Angela, turning you on your side will be more comfortable for you.'	Establish eye contact.	Warm hands.

Transfer from lying to sitting no. 1

ADL:	**Transfer from lying to sitting no. 1 (non-adjustable back rest)**
RTC:	**Grabbing staff**
	Waving arms and legs
	Swearing
	Screaming
	Hitting
	Kicking
Technique:	**Cocooning**
Number of care staff:	**1–2**

Possible triggers of RTC:

■ Lack of security, sensation of falling.
■ Establishing balance.
■ Due to fright or anxiety.
■ Misunderstands the care interaction.

Cocooning involves wrapping the person being attended in a bed sheet or slide sheet during the sitting up process. After the person has been sat upright, the sheet is removed and care continues. Angela and Rachael demonstrate this technique.

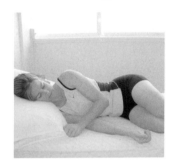

The usual approach used to transfer from lying in bed to sitting on the side of the bed is to position Angela on her side in the lateral or coma position.

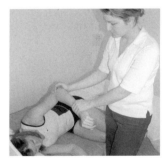

Whilst in the coma (lateral) position if Angela waves her arms and/or grabs at Rachael, Rachael can gently hold Angela's wrist and elbow as shown in the photograph.

Rachael then soothingly and gently strokes Angela's forearm and through conversation relaxes Angela.

4 The Interaction

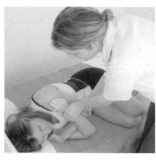

Once Angela is relaxed, Rachael folds Angela's arms into a chest-hugging position.

Rachael talks Angela through the process.

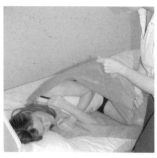

Rachael folds the bed sheet over Angela's upper shoulder and brings the sheet around the front of Angela so that the sheet can be held by Rachael under Angela's lower shoulder near the mattress.

Rachael brings the sheet to Angela's waist only, otherwise it is hard to remove the sheet at the end of the technique and Angela could slide off the bed.

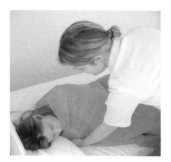

Rachael has now wrapped Angela, snugly, and her arms are contained. With her left hand Rachael continues to hold the linen wrapped around Angela at her shoulder.

Rachael keeps her body positioned between Angela's upper and lower body adjacent to Angela's waist. This is the best point of leverage and reduces the risk of being kicked.

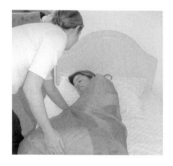

Rachael keeps her hands on Angela's shoulder and places her right hand on Angela's thigh or just above the knee.

Rachael then lowers Angela's legs to the side of the bed. This helps to bring Angela's body up to a seated position on the edge of the bed.

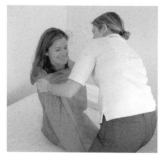

Angela has been sat up on the edge of the bed, and Rachael assists Angela to obtain her sitting balance.

Once Angela is upright Rachael removes the bed sheet, or slide sheet, by pushing it back out of the way. This is important to prevent Rachael or Angela tripping on the bed sheet.

✓ **Key Learning:** Transfer from lying to sitting no. 1		
Contextual communication		**Contextual tasking**
Verbal communication	**Non-verbal communication**	**Third party props**
Explain care activity and purpose and give the person time to adjust to this. Rachael verbally reassures Angela, using words of encouragement.	Rachael holds Angela in the cocooning position, whilst maintaining eye contact.	Warm the room to a temperature comfortable for the person who is undressed. Reduce background noise. Wrap in sheet, drawsheet, slide sheet or incontinence bed sheet.

4 The Interaction

Transfer from lying to sitting no. 2

ADL:	**Transfer from lying to sitting no. 2 (adjustable backrest)**
RTC:	**Grabbing**
	Waving arms and legs
	Swearing
	Screaming
	Hitting
	Kicking
Technique:	**Cocooning**
Number of care staff:	**1–2**

Possible triggers of RTC:

- Lack of security, sensation of falling.
- Establishing balance.
- Due to fright or anxiety.
- Misunderstands the care interaction.

Cocooning involves the wrapping of the person being attended in a bed sheet or slide sheet during the sitting up process. After the person has been sat upright, the sheet is removed and care continues. This technique is demonstrated.

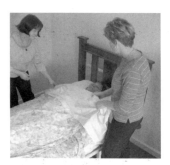

Before transferring, the usual approach is for the care staff member to pull back the bed sheet.

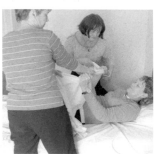

The person responds to being uncovered by grabbing the bed linen and pulling against the care staff.

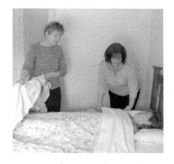

The alternative to pulling linen off the person is to draw the linen up from the bottom of the bed and cocoon the person.

Notice how one care staff member has established eye contact and is engaging the person.

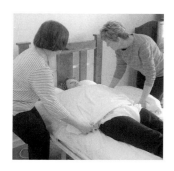

The bed linen is wrapped around the person using the cocoon technique. This means that only half of the person's body is exposed. The bed linen is tucked under her.

Note: only a sheet and blanket should be used. Continental quilts can be too thick and interfere in good manual handling practices.

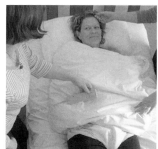

The back of the bed is then raised to sit the person in bed.

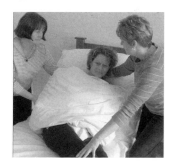

The care staff member then sits the person up onto the side of the bed.

Keeping the person cocooned keeps her warm and prevents her from grabbing.

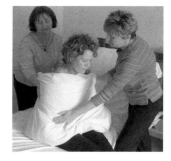

Once the person has been sat upright on the side of the bed, and balanced, the care staff member removes the sheet and blankets.

✓ Key Learning: Transfer from lying to sitting no. 2		
Contextual communication		Contextual tasking
Verbal communication	**Non-verbal communication**	**Third party props**
Explain the care activity and purpose and give the person time to adjust. A care staff verbally reassures the person using words of encouragement.	The care staff holds the person in the cocooning position whilst maintaining eye contact.	Warm room temperature. Warm hands. Reduced background noise. Wrap in sheet and blanket.

4 The Interaction

Mechanical hoist

ADL:	**Full body hoist**
RTC:	**Grabbing fixtures or fittings**
	Waving arms and legs
	Stiffening or rigidity of the body
Technique:	**Chest hugging**
Number of care staff:	**1–2**

Possible triggers of RTC:

- Fear of the unknown.
- Moving from the comfort and safety of bed.
- Being off the ground, fear of falling.
- Unfamiliar activity.
- Misunderstands the interaction.
- Feeling cold or cold environment.

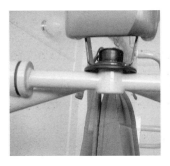 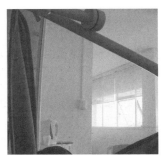

This is the visual field that a person has when sitting in a sling. It does not contextualise the activity.

In a prone position the visual field may be of the arm of the hoist or a wall or window. This view does not orientate the person to the purpose of the care activity.

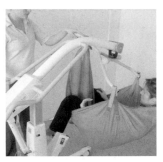

This photograph shows the incorrect technique of facing the person toward the hoist during the transfer.
Note that Angela's feet are hitting the hoist.

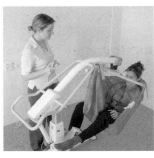

The correct position in the sling for Angela is at right angles to the hoist, which prevents Angela's feet hitting the hoist. But note that Rachael is standing where she can be kicked.

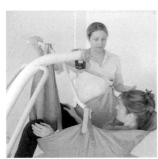

To prevent being kicked Rachael needs to stand to one side of Angela and establish eye contact with her.

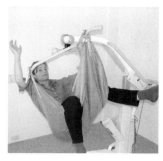

In this position, if Angela panics whilst in the sling, stiffening her body or waving her arms and legs, she will not injure herself or Rachael.

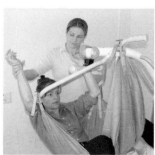

To calm Angela in the hoist, do not approach her from behind as she cannot see you.

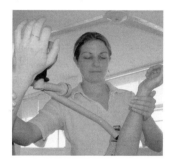

The correct approach is for Rachael to stand to one side where she can have direct eye contact with Angela.

Rachael then gently brings Angela's forearms down to her body into the chest-hugging position.
That is, crossing her arms against her chest.

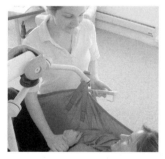

Rachael gently supports Angela's arms in the chest-hugging position with one of her hands and maintains eye contact with her.

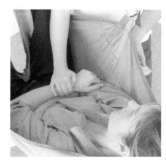

Rachael also verbally reassures Angela during the body lift.

✓ **Key Learning:** Mechanical hoist		
Contextual communication		**Contextual tasking**
Verbal communication	**Non-verbal communication**	**Third party props**
Explain care activity and purpose and give the person time to adjust to this.	Rachael gently holds Angela's forearms in the chest-hugging position and maintains eye contact with her.	Full lighting.
		Warm room temperature.
Rachael verbally reassures Angela using words of encouragement such as, 'Angela, you are safe and secure in this hoist.'	Use non-thumb technique to prevent skin tear.	Quiet environment.
		Hoist/sling correctly positioned.
	If the person is prone to skin tears cover forearms.	

Stand transfer

ADL:	**Stand transfer from sitting**
RTC:	**Grabbing, including staff**
	Waving arms
Technique:	**Cupping hands**
Number of care staff:	**1–2**

Possible triggers of RTC:

■ Misunderstands the care interaction.
■ Visual deficit: despite visual prompts Molly does not see the walking frame.
■ Fear of the unknown.

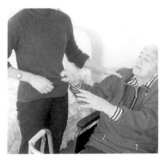

Molly cannot see the walking frame placed in front of her by the care staff member standing by her side.

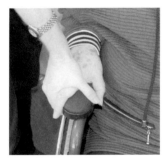

Because Molly does not understand what is happening she grabs Angela's clothing.

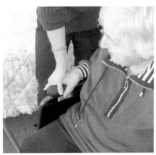

To help Molly do a stand transfer stand in front, where she can see you, establish eye contact and show her the walking frame and explain what you are about to do. Then move to her side and give verbal prompts whilst gently placing one of Molly's hands on the chair or wheelchair armrest.

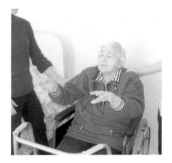

Note that Molly is now looking at her right hand as the care staff member verbally and physically prompts Molly to the action required.

Now place Molly's left hand on the walking frame that is positioned in front of her within easy reaching distance.

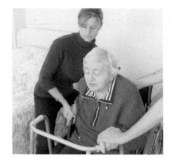

Note that both care staff are now gently securing Molly's hands, one on the armrest for leverage to stand, and one on the walking frame for balance.

Only one care staff member continues talking to Molly to maintain Molly's focus on the transfer.

Continue the stand transfer with both care staff.

✓ **Key Learning:** Stand transfer from sitting		
Contextual communication		**Contextual tasking**
Verbal communication	**Non-verbal communication**	**Third party props**
Explain the care activity and purpose and give the person time to adjust to this.	Physically prompt Molly by showing her where to place her hands: one on the chair and one on the walking frame.	Show the walking frame to the person and place within reach of their chair.
Explain one step of the care activity at a time.		Ensure the person is wearing shoes that are non-slip, fit properly and that laces are tied up, before commencing the transfer.

Correcting sitting posture

ADL:	**Correcting sitting posture**
RTC:	**Pulling away**
	Stiffening body
Technique:	**Upper arm rub**
Number of care staff:	**1–2**

In this scenario the care staff member attempts to sit Molly upright in the armchair. This is made difficult by three factors:

■ Molly is leaning to the right, so her weight is on her right hip and buttock.
■ Molly's bottom is now positioned to off centre in the chair.
■ Molly has adjusted her view of the world and sudden correction of her posture will lead to her pushing in the direction she is leaning (see spatial perception) as Molly has a perceptual deficit.

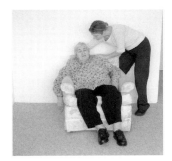

Rachael attempts to pull Molly into the upright position.

However, Molly pulls away because being pulled suddenly from a leaning position to an upright position makes her feel off balance. So Molly resists Rachael.

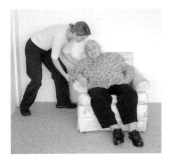

Rachael then attempts to correct Molly's position by pushing Molly into the upright position.

Note that Molly's bottom and legs are off centre, so it will be difficult to move her into a vertical position.

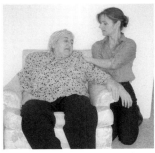

In this photograph Angela has repositioned Molly's feet to be centred to her body.

Angela then rubs Molly's upper arm whilst telling her to lean toward the arm being rubbed.

This technique allows Molly to largely correct her own position.

✓ Key Learning: Correct sitting posture		
Contextual communication		**Contextual tasking**
Verbal communication	**Non-verbal communication**	**Third party props**
Explain the care activity and purpose and give the person time to adjust to this. Verbally prompt the person to correct their own position.	Reposition the person's feet to be centred to her body. Rub the upper arm on the side you want Molly to lean towards.	Use a mirror in front of the person so they can see when they are properly upright.

Wheelchair mobilising

ADL:	**Wheelchair mobilising**
RTC:	**Grabbing fixtures and fittings**
	Pushing back
Technique:	**Chest hugging**
Number of care staff:	**1–2**

Possible triggers for RTC:

■ Misunderstands the care interaction.
■ Does not want to be moved.
■ Deteriorating eyesight affects spatial perception, so thinks that a crash is likely.
■ Wheelchair moving too quickly, causing panic or anxiety.

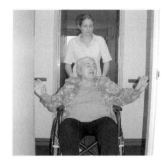

In this photograph Molly has extended both arms with both hands in an attempt to grasp the door frame and door handle.

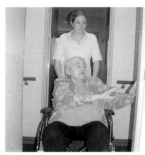

Molly's attention is now focused on the left wall as she reaches for a fixture to grasp. Rachael stops, comes around to the front where Molly can see her, obtains eye contact and explains the care activity about to take place. She asks Molly to cross her arms in the chest-hugging position for her safety.

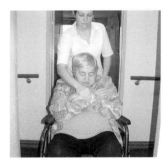

Rachael encourages Molly to look at her hands and arms, to keep her focus on her hands and not the walls or doorway.

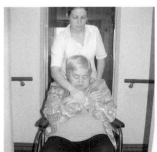

Rachael continues to hold Molly's arms gently and talk to her whilst slowly wheeling her.

Rachael may also offer Molly something to hold to occupy her hands.

4 The Interaction

✓ **Key Learning:** Wheelchair mobilising		
Contextual communication		**Contextual tasking**
Verbal communication	**Non-verbal communication**	**Third party props**
Explain care activity and purpose and give the person time to adjust to this. Continue to provide verbal reassurance.	Physically prompt the person to cross their arms in the chest-hugging position. Hold the person's hands whilst wheeling.	Clear the passage of obstacles if present and wheel the person slowly to the destination. Offer the person something to hold to keep their hands occupied.

Continence pad change – standing

ADL:	**Application of continence pad – standing**
RTC:	**Grabbing**
	Hitting
	Stiffening limbs
Technique:	**Standing pad change**
Number of care staff:	**1–2**

Possible triggers for RTC

■ Misunderstands the care interaction.
■ Feels vulnerable undressed.
■ Becomes cold during the changing of wet pad or clothes.

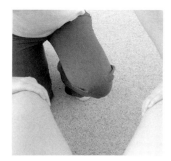

This photo shows that Rachael is forcing Angela's legs apart to fit the pad in place.

DO NOT use this approach to continence management.

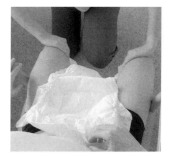

Hips are designed for forward movement only and this technique forces the hip joints to externally rotate, which can be painful to the older person.

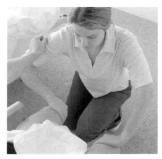

Also, Rachael is in a position where she can be kicked, hit or grabbed by Angela.

4 The Interaction

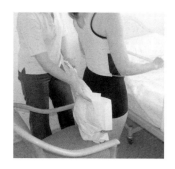

The correct technique is to stand Angela upright.
Rachael stands at Angela's side and provides Angela with a solid handrail to hold.

If a second care staff member is available then this person can support Angela's grasp of the rail and standing position and reassure Angela during the care activity.

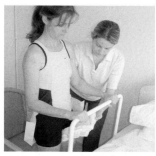

Rachael applies the pad to Angela's buttocks and then draws it through between her legs to the front, fastens it and assists Angela to sit down.

✓ Key Learning: Continence pad change standing		
Contextual communication		**Contextual tasking**
Verbal communication	**Non-verbal communication**	**Third party props**
Explain the care activity and purpose and give the person time to adjust to this.	Physically prompt Angela to stand.	Show the person the clean pad.
Verbally prompt the person with words of encouragement.		Set up the bed rail or other support for the person to hold and balance on.
		Warm room temperature.

Continence pad change in bed no. 1

ADL:	**Continence pad change in bed no. 1**
RTC:	**Grabbing staff**
	Waving arms and legs
	Swearing
	Screaming
	Hitting
	Kicking
Technique:	**Cocooning**
Number of care staff:	**1–2**

Possible triggers of RTC:

■ Lack of security, sensation of falling.
■ Establishing balance.
■ Due to fright or anxiety.
■ Misunderstands the care interaction.

Cocooning involves the wrapping of the person being attended in a bed sheet or slide sheet during the sitting up process. After the person has been sat up, the sheet is removed and care continues. This technique is demonstrated below.

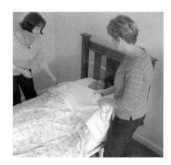

Before changing a continence pad the usual approach is for the care staff to pull back the bed sheet.

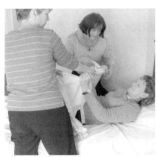

The person responds to being uncovered by grabbing the bed linen and pulling against the care staff.

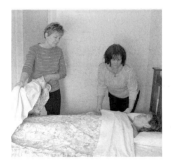

The alternative to pulling linen off the person is to draw the linen up from the bottom of the bed and cocoon the person.

Notice how one care staff member has established eye contact and is engaging the person.

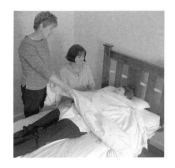

The bed linen is wrapped around the person using the cocoon technique. This means that only half of the person's body is exposed. The bed linen is then tucked under the person.

Note: only a sheet and blanket should be used.
Continental quilts/doonas can be too thick and interfere in good manual handling practices.

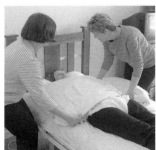

The bed linen is tucked under the person (not the mattress).

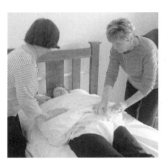

The care staff then change the continence pad. Keeping the person cocooned keeps her warm and prevents her from grabbing.

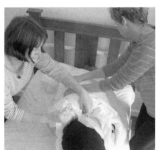

Whilst cocooned it is possible to reposition the person from side to side to allow the change of the pad and hygiene to be maintained.

If cocooning is used frequently then consider leaving the sheet and blankets untucked.

✓ Key Learning: Continence pad change in bed no. 1		
Contextual communication		**Contextual tasking**
Verbal communication	**Non-verbal communication**	**Third party props**
Explain the care activity and purpose and give the person time to adjust.	The care staff holds the person in the cocooning position whilst maintaining eye contact.	Warm room temperature.
		Warm hands.
Verbally reassure the person using words of encouragement and emotive words, e.g. snug and warm.		Reduced background noise.
		Cocoon in sheet and blanket.

4 The Interaction

Continence pad change in bed no. 2

ADL:	**Continence pad change in bed no. 2**
RTC:	**Grabbing**
	Hitting
	Stiffening limbs
	Body rigidity
Technique:	**Holding bed rail**
Number of care staff:	**1–2**

Possible triggers for RTC:

■ Misunderstands the care interaction.
■ Feels vulnerable undressed.
■ Becomes cold during changing of wet pad or clothes.
■ Awoken suddenly.

In this procedure Rachael is applying a continence pad to Angela whilst she lies in bed. If Angela is known to grab at the pad then a second care staff member is required to assist.

Care staff 1 attends the activity of applying the pad.
Care staff 2 engages Angela and supports her grasp of the safety rail.

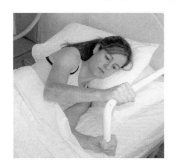

Rachael has positioned Angela to face the raised safety rail. Rachael has placed both of Angela's hands onto the safety rail.

This occupies Angela's attention and her hands, and provides her with a sense of security.

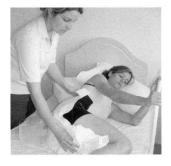

Rachael uncovers Angela and positions the new continence pad, commencing from the back and then bringing it forward.

If there is a second care staff member they should stand opposite Rachael, directly in front of Angela, reassuring her and encouraging Angela to keep hold of the rail.

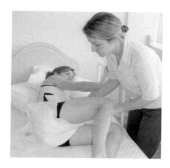

If working alone, Rachael moves to the other side of the bed and positions the pad between Angela's legs, whilst continuing to reassure and ensure that Angela holds onto the safety rail, thereby occupying her hands.

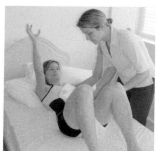

If Angela exhibits RTC, Rachael should stop applying the continence pad and talk to Angela to comfort her and calm her.

Rachael may offer Angela a soft object to hold during the care.

✓ Key Learning: Continence pad change in bed no. 2		
Contextual communication		**Contextual tasking**
Verbal communication	**Non-verbal communication**	**Third party props**
Explain the care activity and purpose and give the person time to adjust to this.	Physically prompt the person's hands to hold the safety rail.	Show the person the dry pad.
	Stop if the person exhibits RTC. Comfort and calm before recommencing care.	Warm the room temperature.
Use verbal prompts to reinforce the care activity such as, 'Angela, this pad is dry. It will be more comfortable and warm for you.'		Dimmed lighting if in the middle of the night.
		Warm hands.
Use reassuring words if Angela exhibits RTC.		

Toileting

ADL:	**Toileting without rails**
RTC:	**Back arching**
	Grabbing
	Hitting
	Stiffening limbs
Technique:	**Body rigidity**
Number of care staff:	**1–2**

Possible triggers of RTC:

■ Sense of falling.
■ Cool, uncomfortable room temperature.
■ Misunderstands the care activity.
■ Nothing to hold onto for security.
■ Feeling vulnerable undressed.

Toileting without rails

Sitting on a toilet requires the same physical ability as sitting on a chair, but is made more complex by the lower height of the toilet compared to a chair and no side hand rails to hold on to.

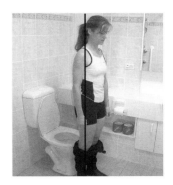

Angela illustrates the common upright posture prior to sitting on the toilet.

The line marks her centre of gravity.

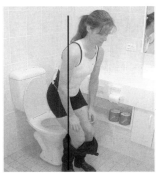

Angela illustrates how far from the centre of gravity (stable standing base) a person has to counter-balance to be able to sit over a toilet.

4 The Interaction

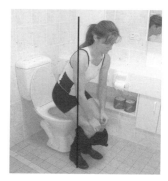

The natural technique to sitting on a toilet is to counter-balance the buttocks as they push out over the toilet. A squatting action is used by bending the knees and leaning forward, thereby moving the torso forward.

This action keeps the weight evenly distributed over the stable standing base.

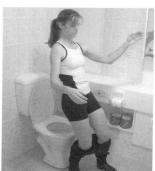

In this photograph Angela demonstrates that if she does not bend at the hips it makes it extremely difficult for her to sit on the toilet.

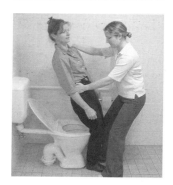

Rachael shows that if Angela stiffens, her centre of balance is lost and her weight pulls away from her.

Rachael attempts to counter-balance Angela's weight by bending her knees and holding her own weight back.

DO NOT do this.

Continuing to attempt to position a person on to the toilet, who becomes rigid during the transfer, is likely to result in injury.

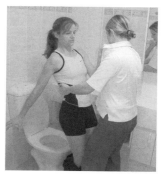

Angela mimics losing her balance and grabs Rachael by the blouse.

Angela is now on the verge of falling and if she does Rachael may also sustain a back injury by attempting to stop her from falling.

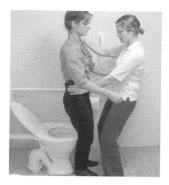

The correct technique is for Rachael to support Angela's upper body with one hand, by holding her shoulder, whilst using her other hand to push down on Angela's hip, to encourage her to bend at the hip and sit down.

Toileting with rails

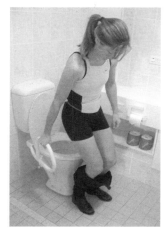

Angela shows how a toilet seat armrest allows her to maintain stability, similar to sitting in a chair, as she is able to place her weight on the side armrests.

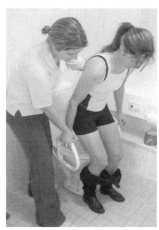

Rachael can then assist Angela from the side. Rachael places her left hand on Angela's left shoulder, with the forearm resting down Angela's back, to apply a stable slightly backward and downward pressure to Angela's shoulder. This assists Angela to bend at the waist.

Rachael's right hand is supporting Angela's right hand that is gripping the toilet armrest.

To prevent Angela's feet slipping forward, Rachael could place her right foot at a right angle in front of Angela's feet.

Toileting using a shower chair

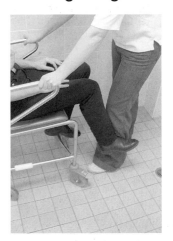

In this position Rachael can be kicked by Angela.

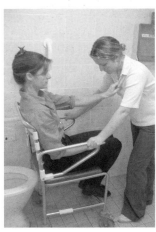

In this position Rachael's shirt or body can be grabbed, hit or pinched by Angela.

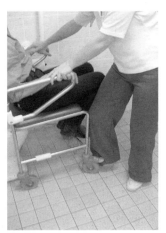

Rachael positions the shower chair castors so that they are aligned to roll directly backwards.

Rather than standing in front of the chair Rachael positions herself to one side so she can't be kicked.

Rachael uses her right knee to help position the shower chair, that is, to increase the forward thrust over the toilet.

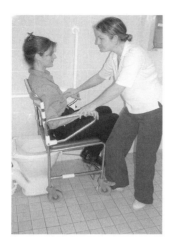

To prevent being grabbed Rachael supports Angela's grip of the armrests of the shower chair by placing her own hands over Angela's hands.

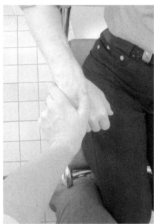

Notice that the heel/butt of Rachael's hand is resting against the shower chair armrest and is not pushing onto Angela's hand.

✓ **Key Learning:** Toileting

Contextual communication		Contextual tasking
Verbal communication	**Non-verbal communication**	**Third party props**
Explain the care activity and purpose and give the person time to adjust to this.	Physically prompt the person's hands to the correct position	Well lit bathroom.
		Warm bathroom temperature.
		Place a towel over the person's lap for privacy.

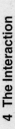

4 The Interaction

Showering

ADL:	**Showering**
RTC:	**Grabbing soft items**
	Grabbing fixtures and fittings
	Grabbing care staff
	Yelling
Technique:	**Facing the person toward the care staff member**
Number of care staff:	**1–2**

Possible triggers of RTC:

■ Bathroom temperature is cooler than bedroom.
■ Noise from the fan may cause fright/panic, or interfere with hearing.
■ Voice echo may cause confusion.
■ Feel vulnerable undressed.
■ Misunderstands the care interaction.

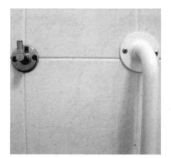

This photograph shows the view a person sees if faced toward the shower wall.

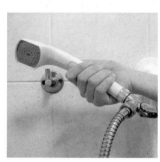

A shower rose suddenly appearing squirting water will probably frighten or confuse the person.

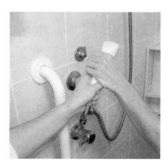

A common RTC behaviour in this situation is the person grabbing the shower rose from the care staff member.

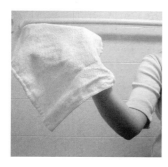

Approaching the person's face with an open face flannel can partially or fully obscure the person's visual field, which can also frighten and confuse.

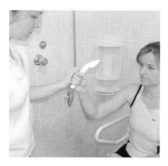

Angela demonstrates the natural reaction for the person whose visual field is suddenly blocked – she grabs the face flannel.

The next five photographs illustrate specific techniques designed to engage the person in the shower.

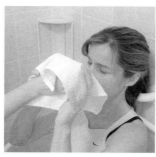

It is preferable that the person being showered faces out toward the care staff rather than to the wall (if safe to do so). Angela can now see Rachael, the shower rose, and the face flannel. Rachael explains the interaction to Angela, using repetitive key words like 'shower', 'water' and 'wash' to help Angela understand the care interaction being carried out.

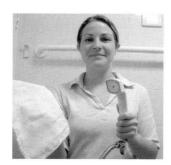

Rachael offers Angela the shower rose to hold to promote independence and participation, if it is safe to do so.

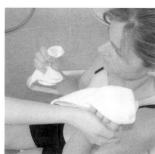

Rachael offers Angela a face flannel and assists Angela by guiding her hand to bring the face flannel to her own body.

4 The Interaction

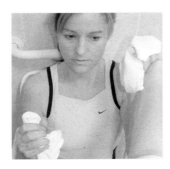

Angela demonstrates how, even when she can't wash herself, she still prefers to hold a face flannel.

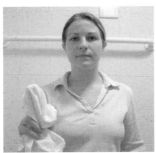

Rachael demonstrates the approach to washing Angela's face in which she has wrapped the face flannel over three of her fingers so Angela's visual field is not obscured by the face flannel.

✓　**Key Learning:**　Showering

Contextual communication		Contextual tasking
Verbal communication	**Non-verbal communication**	**Third party props**
Explain the care activity and purpose and give the person time to adjust to this. Reinforce purpose using key words such as, 'Angela, it is time for your shower. The water will be warm. You enjoy having a warm shower.'	Face the person outwardly, from recess if possible. Once undressed wrap towels around shoulders and torso and across the person's lap for privacy and warmth. Check water temperature is warm and wet person's feet first, working up the body. Do not spray water directly onto the person's face.	Warm temperature. If the person walks in the bathroom place bath mat(s) or towels on the floor so it is not cold and wet under foot. Place items on shelf next to the person, e.g. soap, shampoo, face washer, to help orientate them to the purpose of the activity. Dress warmly prior to leaving the bathroom to accommodate for the cooler bedroom.

4　The Interaction

Dressing

ADL:	**Dressing**
RTC:	**Chest hugging**
	Grabbing soft items
Technique:	**Threading**
Number of care staff:	**1–2**

Possible triggers of RTC:

■ Misunderstands the care interaction.
■ Sight deficit.
■ Fear of the unknown.
■ Not wanting to get dressed.
■ Movement of contracted limb causing pain.

Commence dressing – use the arm with the least range of movement.
Commence undressing – use the arm with the greatest range of movement.

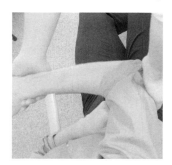

Rachael places one hand under Angela's elbow and the other hand under Angela's wrist. Rachael then supports and gently rotates Angela's shoulder within its range of movement diagonally across Angela's body. This frees up Angela's arm to commence dressing.

DO NOT pull Angela's arm directly up and/or out.

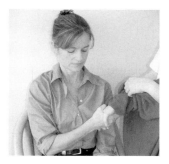

Rachael turns the cardigan inside out by rolling it back onto her own arm. To dress Angela, Rachael stands diagonally opposite the arm she is attending. When dressing the right arm Rachael stands on Angela's left side.

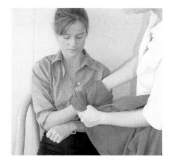

When Rachael rolls the cardigan onto Angela's arm the cardigan will be the right way out. This is called threading.

Notice how Angela is clearly focused on the dressing process. This focus is reinforced by Rachael speaking about the process in simple steps throughout the care interaction.

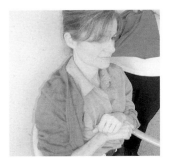

Rachael then brings the cardigan around Angela's right shoulder, across the top of her back to above her left shoulder.

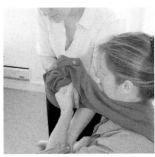

Rachael then moves across to Angela's right side so she can dress her left arm, always approaching on a diagonal.

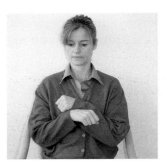

In the final step Rachael pulls the cardigan down Angela's back, adjusts the sleeves on the cardigan and buttons the cardigan.

The technique, threading, can be used with most garments.

✓ **Key Learning:** Dressing		
Contextual communication		**Contextual tasking**
Verbal communication	**Non-verbal communication**	**Third party props**
Explain the care activity and purpose and give the person time to adjust to this.	Stand diagonally and on the opposite side of the limb you want to dress.	Warm hands.
Reinforce the purpose using key words such as, 'Angela, this is your cardigan. Your cardigan will keep you warm. You like being warm.'	Establish eye contact when explaining the activity.	Show the person the cardigan.

Putting shoes on

ADL:	**Putting shoes on**
RTC:	**Kicking**
	Hair pulling
Technique:	**Side position and leg raise**
Number of care staff:	**1**

Possible triggers of RTC:

- Discomfort experienced as shoe is applied.
- Intrusion on personal space.
- Misunderstands the care interaction.

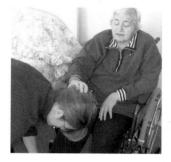

In this photograph Angela is putting Molly's shoe on and has positioned herself directly in front, within reach of Molly. In this position Molly is able to grab and pull Angela's hair.

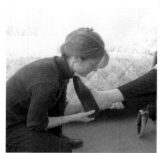

This photograph shows Angela squatting directly in front of Molly. In this position Molly is able to kick Angela in the face.

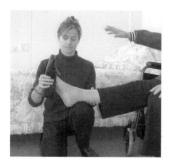

The correct technique is for Angela to position herself out of Molly's reach, then place Molly's foot on her knee to put the shoe on.

Angela could also use a stool to support Molly's leg.

This should be performed within the person's range of movment and should NOT be performed on a person where it is medically contraindicated, e.g. someone who has had a recent hip replacement.

4 The Interaction

✓ Key Learning: Putting shoes on		
Contextual communication		**Contextual tasking**
Verbal communication	**Non-verbal communication**	**Third party props**
Explain the care activity you are about to undertake. Give the person time to take this in. Repeat key words to reinforce the activity such as, 'Angela, these are your shoes. Your shoes keep your feet warm and comfortable.'	Make eye contact, and point to the person's shoe and foot. Squat to one side and out of arm's reach.	Show the person the shoes. Ensure the footwear is the correct size and fit.

Assisting to eat

ADL:	**Assisting to eat**
RTC:	**Turning away**
	Refusing to open mouth
Technique:	**Rooting and suck reflexes**
Number of care staff:	**1**

Possible triggers of RTC:

- The person is not being assisted to eat in a way that makes sense to them.
- The person is not aware that it is mealtime.
- Lack of appetite.
- The food looks or smells unfamiliar.
- Misunderstands the care interaction.
- Does not know what kind of food it is.

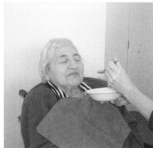

In this photograph Molly is being offered food on a spoon. The care staff member, spoon and bowl of food are clearly visible to Molly.

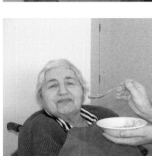

However, Molly keeps closing her eyes and mouth and turning her face away when Rachael brings a spoon of food to Molly's mouth.

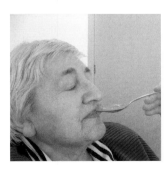

Rachael attempts to stimulate the suck reflex by placing a small amount of food on Molly's top lip.

However, Molly keeps her eyes and mouth closed.

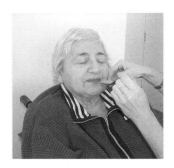

Rachael then stimulates the rooting reflex by stimulating Molly's left cheek, but Molly continues to keep her eyes and mouth closed.

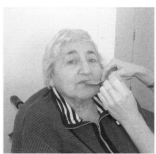

Rachael uses verbal prompts by describing the food, its taste and smell, and stimulates both the rooting and suck reflexes. Molly opens her eyes and mouth and tastes the food.

✓ Key Learning:	Assisting to eat	
Contextual communication		**Contextual tasking**
Verbal communication	**Non-verbal communication**	**Third party props**
Explain the care activity and purpose and give the person time to adjust to this.	Sit where the person can see you and the spoon and bowl of food.	Serviette or napkin on their lap.
Use key words to reinforce the purpose of the activity and to stimulate appetite. 'Molly, the chicken soup is warm and tasty. It smells great. You like chicken soup.'	Assist the person at their pace.	Eating utensils and plate or bowl on placemat on table in front of them. Aroma of food.

Eating

ADL:	**Defining the eating area**
RTC:	**Taking food from other plates**
Technique:	**Defining the eating area**
Number of care staff:	**1**

Possible triggers of RTC:

- The person thinks that all food on the table is theirs.
- The food on another plate looks different/more interesting.

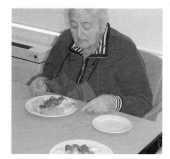

Molly has food on a plate in front of her and has started eating.

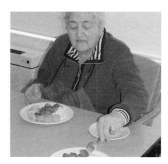

Molly then sees the other plate of food and takes some food from the plate.

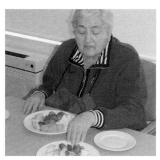

Molly pulls the other plate toward her to pick off some food.

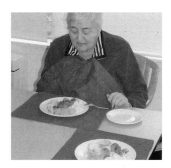

Defining the personal space using contrasting coloured props focuses Molly on her food as it helps identify her personal space. This can be done by contrasting the colours of the food and plate, the plate and placemat, and contrasting the placemat from the table.

✓ Key Learning: Defining the eating area		
Contextual communication		**Contextual tasking**
Verbal communication	**Non-verbal communication**	**Third party props**
Explain the purpose of the dining room and type of meal to the person.	Focus the person's attention on the condiments, food and table setting	Place the plate of food directly in front of the person.
Name the food for the person.		Put a placemat that is a different colour to the table under the plate.
Use verbal prompts to help the person focus on the meal.		Place eating utensils on the placemat.
Avoid discussing topics other than the meal.		Place a serviette or napkin on the person's lap.
		Well lit dining room.
		Soft music playing or quiet environment.
		Aroma of food.

Sundowning

RTC:	**Sundowning**
Technique:	**Validate and distract**
Number of care staff:	**1**

Sundowning is when the person with dementia experiences an acute increase in disorientation or deterioration in cognition, with a sudden onset of restlessness and confusion, in the late afternoon into the early evening.

Possible triggers of RTC:

- Lack of sensory stimulation, e.g. lower lighting in the evening.
- Tiredness.
- Background noise.
- Frustration with activities of daily living and social and recreational activities.
- Increased misinterpretation of events.
- Seeking security and emotional warmth.
- Hunger.

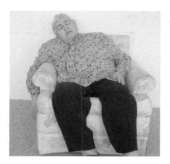

Molly has sat herself in a chair and has been crying, calling for her mother.

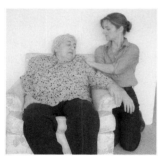

Angela responds by comforting Molly and uses the validate and distract technique to calm her.

Molly:	'I want my mum she's not home.' (upset)
Care staff member:	'Its okay Molly . . . you miss your mum?' (reassuring tone and touch)
Molly:	'Yes, I want my mum.' (upset)
Care staff member:	'She's a good mum.' (reassuring tone and touch)
Molly:	'Yes, she should be here.' (worried)
Care staff member:	'It's almost tea time . . . Is your mum a good cook?' (distract)
Molly:	'Yes.'
Care staff member:	'Does she cook roasts?' (distract)
Molly:	'Yes, roasts.'
Care staff member:	'And her gravy, does she make nice gravy?'
Molly:	'Yes, good gravy.'
Care staff member:	'And dessert, what about apple pie?' (distract)
Molly:	'Mmmm.'

4 The Interaction

✓ **Key Learning:** Sundowning		
Contextual communication		**Contextual tasking**
Verbal communication	**Non-verbal communication**	**Third party props**
Speak calmly and reinforce the person's positive feelings.	Eye contact.	Items that reinforce the positive distraction, in the example given, would be taking her to the kitchen, offering her food and looking at the menu.
Encourage the person to speak.	Gentle touch.	
Use verbal positive distraction. This means moving the person's thoughts away from feelings of loss or grief to happier memories.	Listening.	
Avoid telling lies, such as assuring Molly that her mother is coming soon and avoid reality orientation, such as telling Molly that her mother is dead.		

Catastrophic reaction

RTC:	**Catastrophic reaction**
Technique:	**Diagonal approach**
Number of care staff:	**1**

Catastrophic reactions are an over-reaction to a minor stress.

Possible triggers of RTC:

- Losing or misplacing items.
- Cognitive overload, too much stimuli.
- Inability to perform a task.
- Fatigue.
- Misinterpretation of sensory information, e.g. misunderstanding another person's posture or non-verbal communication.
- Inability to communicate needs and/or being misunderstood.

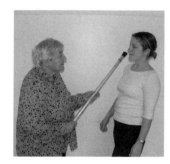

In this photograph Rachael has asked Molly to come to the toilet. Molly has responded with a catastrophic reaction, hitting Rachael in the face and yelling at Rachael.

The incorrect technique is for Rachael to raise her voice and tell Molly to relax.

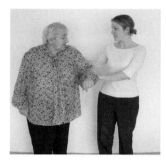

The correct approach is for Rachael is to increase Molly's personal space by moving away from Molly until the emotion subsides, then slowly approach from a diagonal or side position.

Rachael also acknowledges and validates Molly's emotion. Catastrophic reactions can be tiring for the person with dementia so the aim is to minimise the extent of the reaction.

✓	**Key Learning:** Catastrophic reaction		
	Contextual communication		**Contextual tasking**
	Verbal communication	**Non-verbal communication**	**Third party props**
	Speak calmly and slowly to the person so they have time to understand what is being said.	Calmly and slowly approach the person diagonally from the front.	Reduce background noise.
	Validate the person's emotion.	Establish eye contact.	
	Find out what the person needs.	Keep hands by your side.	
		Keep a reasonable distance from the person until they have calmed. Then touch to reassure.	

Wandering

RTC:	**Walking away**
	Pulling away
Technique:	**Diagonal approach**
Number of care staff:	**1**

Possible triggers of RTC:

- Uncertain about their own needs.
- Pre-illness habitual behaviours, such as the person who always took a walk before breakfast.
- Long-term memory driven behaviours.
- The person is going somewhere or looking for something, even if we do not know what it is.
- Delusion driven walking, such as the person who feels they are in a concentration camp or gaol.
- Other causes, such as medical issues, e.g. pain, cerebral irritation, continence issues.

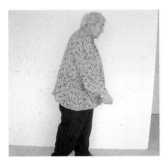

This photograph shows Molly wandering and she has become tired and irritable.

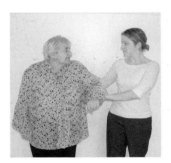

The correct approach is for Rachael to approach Molly using a diagonal approach so as not to frighten Molly, and then move to her side.

Notice how Rachael and Molly now have direct eye contact and Rachael holds Molly's forearm gently using the forearm placement technique. Rachael is now able to validate Molly's emotion and find out what she needs.

✓ **Key Learning:** Wandering		
Contextual communication		**Contextual tasking**
Verbal communication	**Non-verbal communication**	**Third party props**
Speak calmly and reinforce the person's positive feelings.	Calmly and slowly approach the wandering person diagonally from the front. The approach is less intimidating to the person.	Items that reinforce the positive distraction, such as offering food and drink.
Encourage the person to speak.		Involve Molly in an activity that she likes, e.g. folding napkins, watching a video of the family.
User positive verbal distraction. This means moving the person's thoughts away from wandering to another activity.	Establish eye contact. Gently touch using forearm placement technique.	
	Listening.	

Hitting – standing

RTC:	**Hitting**
	Slapping
Technique:	**Forearm placement technique**
Number of care staff:	**1**

Possible triggers of RTC:

■ Incorrectly approaching a person who is agitated.
■ The person feels threatened by the care staff member.

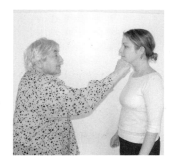

Molly is agitated and Rachael has responded by walking directly up and close to Molly.

Molly has responded to Rachael's sudden approach by hitting Rachael.

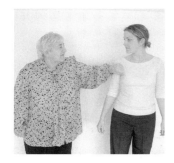

The correct technique is for Rachael to approach Molly from diagonally in front then move to the side. If Molly attempts to hit Rachael the hit will have less accuracy, strength and effect.

Approaching from the diagonal front and then standing to one side is also less threatening to Molly.

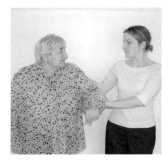

Rachael then responds to Molly by placing one hand on Molly's left elbow and the other on Molly's left wrist.

Using the forearm placement technique makes it very difficult for Molly to hit or strike at Rachael.

✓ **Key Learning:** Hitting – standing

Contextual communication		Contextual tasking
Verbal communication	**Non-verbal communication**	**Third party props**
Speak calmly and reassure the person that they are safe and who you are.	Approach the person slowly from the diagonal front then move to the side.	Quiet environment. Item to occupy them in their hands, e.g. handbag, clothing or other soft item.
Find out what they need.	Establish eye contact when explaining the activity.	
	Gentle use of forearm placement technique to prevent being hit.	

Hitting – squatting

RTC: Hitting – squatting
Technique: Forearm placement technique
Number of care staff: 1

Possible triggers of RTC:

- Approaching a person who is agitated and suspicious.
- The person feels threatened by the care staff.

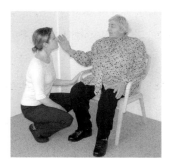

This photograph shows Rachael squatting at face level with Molly.

Molly has responded to Rachael's approach by hitting Rachael in the face.

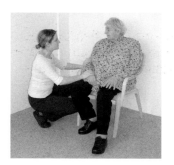

The correct technique is for Rachael to approach Molly by placing one hand on Molly's right elbow and the other on Molly's right wrist before squatting and establishing eye contact with Molly.

Using the forearm placement technique makes it very difficult for Molly to hit or strike out at Rachael.

✓ **Key Learning:** Hitting – squatting

Contextual communication		Contextual tasking
Verbal communication	**Non-verbal communication**	**Third party props**
Speak calmly and reassure the person that they are safe and who you are. Find out what they need.	Establish eye contact and smile to reassure. Gentle use of forearm placement technique to prevent being hit.	Soft items to occupy their hands, e.g. handbag, cloth football or clothing item.

Throwing

RTC: **Throwing**
Technique: **Moving away**
Number of care staff: 1

Possible triggers of RTC:

- Incorrectly approaching a person who is agitated and suspicious.
- The person feels threatened by the care staff member.
- Misunderstands the care interaction.

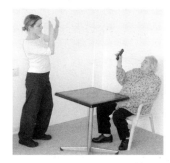

In this photograph Molly is agitated. She has been calling out for help.

Molly has responded to Rachael's approach by picking up the television remote control to throw it at her.

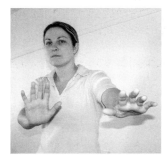

Rachael demonstrates the incorrect response to this situation. Rachael steps forward and reaches for the remote control. This increases the threat to Molly, who is more likely to throw the item.

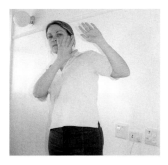

In this photograph Rachael demonstrates the correct response. Rachael steps back, initially guarding her face in case Molly throws the remote control.

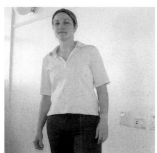

Rachael then lowers her arms and stands in a non-threatening manner to talk and calm Molly.

Once Molly is calm, Rachael approaches slowly, squats down to her level and uses the forearm placement technique to prevent Molly hitting or throwing items.

✓ Key Learning: Throwing		
Contextual communication		**Contextual tasking**
Verbal communication	**Non-verbal communication**	**Third party props**
Speak calmly and reassure the person as to who you are and what you are doing. Find out what they need.	Approach the person slowly from the diagonal front, then squat down to their level. Establish eye contact when explaining the activity. Smile, or show that you are happy to see them.	Quiet environment. Item to occupy them in their hands, e.g. handbag, clothing or other soft item.

Appendix

1. Behavioural reporting
2. Physical and temporal environmental audit
3. Questions and answers:
   - Module 1: Introduction
   - Module 2: The person
   - Module 3: The care staff
   - Module 4: The environment
   - Module 5: The interaction

Appendix 1

Behavioural reporting

The RTC behavioural observation form is a pro forma for behavioural observation of resistance to care. This behavioural observation tool was designed for use in care homes to assist staff to collect observational information to be used to interpret the behaviour of the person with dementia. This observation form should not be used in isolation, but incorporated with other information gained from clinical notes, medical information, family interviews and other nursing and allied health records.

It is recommended that observations be undertaken for a minimum of three days, but preferably five to seven days, to obtain a behavioural overview of the person with dementia.

It is preferable that the recording of observations be made by the person providing the care, e.g. the direct care worker, registered nurse. The evaluation of the behavioural data should be undertaken by suitably qualified health care professionals, e.g. registered nurse, psychiatric nurse, medical officer, who have the necessary expertise to interpret the observations, and then develop and implement a plan of care.

RTC Behavioural Observation Form

Person's name _____   DOB _____   Room number _____
Dates of observation _____

Date & time	Care activity & location (precursor)	Person's response	Duration of behaviour (minutes)	RTC rating (see below)	Describe intervention used & effectiveness	Staff initials & designation

EXAMPLE ONLY

Date & time	Care activity & location (precursor)	Person's response	Duration of behaviour (minutes)	RTC rating	Describe intervention used & effectiveness	Staff initials & designation
5/5/03 8.45 am	Transferred Molly onto the shower chair	Molly grabbed safety rail on bed and would not let go	3	3	Gently stroked the back of Molly's hand and talked about her family. Molly let go.	MH, RN JG, Care Assist.

Rating 1: Mild RTC

■ Agitation that occurs on commencement or during care
■ Confusion that occurs on commencement or during care
■ Incoherence, that occurs on commencement or during care
■ Indifference, not responding to requests
■ Mild verbal non-acceptance
■ Noisy
■ Pulling away just prior to care
■ Not opening the mouth or swallowing
■ Restless
■ Turning away or walking away
■ Unsteady, onset during care
■ Withdrawal

Rating 2: Semi-moderate RTC

■ Grabbing soft items, e.g. towel, clothes, flannel
■ Limbs and/or body going limp
■ Making verbal threats at normal volume
■ Requiring repeated instruction or distraction
■ Slouching into chair or bed
■ Spitting, e.g. out food or medication
■ Swearing or expressing angry non-compliance
■ Verbally objecting to care using words or sounds, e.g. growling
■ Posturing

Rating 3: Moderate RTC

■ Crossing limbs
■ Chest hugging
■ Grabbing staff
■ Grabbing or holding onto fixtures, e.g. chair, bed or hand-rail
■ Making verbal threats at high volume including shouting, screaming, or other strong or violent outbursts of hostility
■ Pulling away during care
■ Pushing
■ Ceasing to weight bear during care
■ Spontaneous rigidity of body or limbs
■ Stiffening limbs
■ Waving arms and legs

Rating 4: Severe RTC

■ Biting
■ Deliberately thwarting care
■ Hitting
■ Kicking
■ Pinching
■ Scratching
■ Slapping
■ Striking or lashing out
■ Strong or physical acts thwarting care
■ Throwing items

Appendix 2

Physical and temporal environmental audit

This Dementia specific environmental audit has been designed for use by a person with a base level understanding of the needs of the person with dementia. The audit is designed to assist staff to identify opportunities to improve the aesthetic and functional aspects of the living environment. It is anticipated that the results of this audit be referred to a committee, within the care home, for consideration of issues identified and development of strategies. The audit should be conducted in reference to Chapter 3 The environment.

This audit is not for use in determining building compliancy with building codes, fire safety, health regulations and other legislative and regulatory requirements.
The environment is comprised of two related elements:

- Physical
- Temporal

The physical environment refers specifically to the impact building design, materials, colours, climate, lighting and odour have on the person with dementia and others working, living and/or visiting.

The temporal environment refers to the impact people, such as those working and living with, or visiting, have on the person with dementia. An example is cleaning routines and their associated noise.

The environmental audit tool is designed to assist in the evaluation of the environment for the person with dementia by drawing together elements of the physical and temporal environments.

Using the environmental audit

The dementia specific environment aims to be sensitive to each person's needs, in consideration of their stage of dementia. Therefore, a dementia specific evaluation of the environment must incorporate sensitivity to each person's:

- Memory
- Cognition, including problem solving
- Language
- Activities of daily living
- Coordination skills and physical ability
- Mood and behaviour

Environmental audit

Contents

Environmental audit

Audit for a specific older person

Person's name _____

Room number _____

Unit _____

General audit

Unit _____

Date _____

Time _____

Auditors names	Position	Signature	Date

Environmental audit

Unit _____ Date _____ Time of day _____

Issue	Yes	No	Potential actions
1. Bathroom – toilet *Climate* ■ Is the bath area warmer than adjacent and public areas, 21–27°C? ■ Can the bathroom temperature be regulated to meet the person's warmth needs? *Visual perception* ■ Are standard sized light switches used that have a contrasting colour to the wall? ■ Are light switches at shoulder height for easy access? ■ Are heat lamps or bathroom lights positioned so that they do not create glare off shiny white tiles or off the floor? ■ Are there sensor lights in the bathroom? *Odour/smell* ■ Is the bathroom fragrant and fresh smelling? *Hearing* ■ Is the bathroom environment quiet, e.g. fan noise, echo? *Accessibility* ■ Is there an adjustable shower rose in the bathroom? ■ Does the toilet seat colour contrast with the toilet base and floor? ■ Are bathmats used on the tiled floor when the person walks barefooted? ■ Is there a grab rail in the shower recess and bathroom area? ■ Is there sufficient shelving space in the shower recess for personal belongings, e.g. soap, powder, shampoo, conditioner, face washer? ■ Are there lever taps in the bathroom? ■ Is the mirror positioned so that the person can sit at the hand basin and see themself?			

Environmental audit

Unit _____ Date _____ Time of day _____

Issue	Yes	No	Potential actions
2. Orientation to own room The main purpose of corridors and passages is to facilitate movement from one place of purpose to another. The corridor and passage need to assist the person to locate their room. *Climate* ■ Is the temperature in the room warm, preferably between 19–24°C. *Visual perception* ■ Can the person see the door sign on their door? ■ Does the person recognise their own room? ■ Is the signage on the door a combination of the person's name with a photo or other familiar object? ■ Is the name on the door the name the person relates to and responds to? ■ Is the light switch at shoulder height for easy access? ■ Is the light switch a different or contrasting colour to the surrounding wall? *Odour/smell* ■ Is the room fragrant and fresh smelling? *Hearing* ■ If the person enjoys music, is it played in their room on a regular basis? *Accessibility* ■ Is the bedroom door a different or contrasting colour to the adjacent walls in the corridor? ■ Would the person find it easier to use lever action door handles? ■ Is the floor a consistent colour and pattern between the room and the corridor?			

Environmental audit

Unit _____ Date _____ Time of day _____

Issue	Yes	No	Potential actions

3. Orientation within own room
The bedroom has multiple purposes but primarily acts as a personal space belonging to the person. The bedroom may be used for rest, relaxation, entertainment of visitors and private activities.
 	
Climate
 	
Is the temperature suitable for the person?
Does the person like having their windows open?
 	
Visual perception
 	
■ Is the furniture in the room familiar to them and suited to their physical ability?
■ Is the person's room personalised with their choice of:
  ■ quilt cover
  ■ photographs and art on walls
  ■ at least one piece of art or photograph on a cupboard that the person lying on their side in bed can see
  ■ a familiar piece of clothing on the bed that is theirs
■ Does the light switch contrast with the wall colour?
■ Is the light switch at shoulder height to assist access?
■ Are there curtains or blinds on windows to reduce or prevent glare from sunlight?
■ Are there task lights in the room, such as bed or floor lamps for night time?
 	
Odour/smell
 	
■ Is the room fresh and/or fragrant smelling?
■ Are favourite or familiar scents used in the room to help the person identify their own room?
 	
Hearing
 	
■ Is the music that is played in the room enjoyable and/or relaxing to the person?
 	
Accessibility
 	
■ Does the colour of the bedroom door contrast with other adjacent doors and adjacent walls?
■ Are there lever action door handles on the door?
■ Is there consistency in floor colour and design/pattern from the room into the corridor?
■ If there is a mat on the floor, is it non-slip?
■ Is the room clear of obstacles or trip hazards on the floor?
■ Is the wardrobe hanging rack at the height of the person, so they can easily reach their clothes?
■ Are commonly used items within reach, e.g. reading glasses, shoes, call bell?
■ Is there a clear passage from the bed to the toilet or commode?			

Environmental audit

Unit _____ Date _____ Time of day _____

Issue	Yes	No	Potential actions
4. Orientation to dining room The main purpose of the dining room is for eating meals, which may include socialising. Some dining rooms are also used for other purposes, such as an activities area and as a combined dining-lounge room. *Climate* ■ Is the temperature comfortable for the person? *Visual perception* ■ Are there visual food props or picture cues that reinforce the purpose of the area as one of eating meals and socialising? ■ Are there placemats under plates that define the person's eating area? ■ Is there task lighting over tables at mealtimes to assist the person in seeing the food and other items on the table? *Odour/smell* ■ Can food aromas be smelt in the dining room, to stimulate appetite? ■ Do care staff describe the food to increase appetite and orientation for the person, including the visually impaired person? *Hearing* ■ Is soft classical background music that the person enjoys used to enhance the dining experience? ■ Is the environment at mealtimes peaceful and/or quiet? *Accessibility* ■ Does the colour of the food contrast with the plate? ■ Does the colour of the plate contrast with the placemat? ■ Does the placemat contrast with the colour of the table? ■ Are placemats that have flower patterns (flowers are meant to be picked) or busy patterns removed from all tables? ■ Are tables that seat four people provided in the dining room? ■ Are there tables where only one or two people can sit?			

Environmental audit

Unit _____ Date _____ Time of day _____

Issue	Yes	No	Potential actions
5. Orientation to kitchen The main purpose of the kitchen is the preparation of meals, cleaning up after meals, followed by socialising and/or therapy programs for the person. *Climate* ■ Is the temperature comfortable for the person? *Visual perception* ■ Does the kitchen area have cues or props that reinforce the purpose of the area as one of food preparation and cleaning up? ■ Is there task lighting over benches and sinks to assist the person in seeing the food and other items on the bench and in the sink? ■ Do the crockery and cooking dishes contrast with the bench? *Odour/smell* ■ Are there food aromas at mealtimes to help stimulate the appetite and assist orientation? *Hearing* ■ During cooking activities with the person, are verbal prompts given for each step of the process? ■ Is background noise reduced so that it is not a distraction? *Accessibility* ■ Has a risk assessment of the kitchen been undertaken? ■ hot water temperature control valve ■ electrical and gas isolation of all appliances ■ coded microwave ovens to prevent use when unsupervised ■ an over-ride switch to control dishwasher ■ isolation of poisons ■ increased lighting over task areas ■ use of crockery with a safety rating ■ secure sharp items until supervised ■ an audible alarm on the refrigerator door to indicate that it has been left open longer than 90 seconds ■ Are small portions of food and fluid available during the activity session to snack on? ■ Are familiar items left in the kitchen, such as tea towels, dish rack, safe cooking utensils, e.g. wooden spoons? ■ Is clutter on the kitchen benches reduced during the activity?			

Environmental audit

Unit _____ Date _____ Time of day _____

Issue	Yes	No	Potential actions
6. Orientation to lounge room The main purpose of the lounge room is for socialising, which can involve passive activities, such as sitting quietly, reading, watching television and listening to music, or it may involve participative activities, such as talking and therapy programs. *Climate* ■ Is the temperature comfortable for the person? *Visual perception* ■ Is there artwork within the lounge room to reinforce the purpose of the area and provide items of interest for care staff to talk to the person about? ■ Are there activities for the person to be engaged in? ■ Is there task or increased lighting over chairs and tables where activities are carried out? *Odour/smell* ■ Are aromatherapy and essential oils used to stimulate or relax? ■ Is the lounge room fresh or fragrant smelling? *Hearing* ■ Do care staff help orientate the person by talking about the comfort of the room, the view from the window, the type of art on the walls and/or the activities underway in the room? ■ Is soft classical or other music played for relaxation? ■ Is the TV or radio in the room at a comfortable hearing volume? ■ If the ambience of the room is a peaceful one do care staff and others avoid calling out? *Accessibility* ■ Are there individual activities available for the person who is looking for something to do? ■ Is there seating arrangement for two or more people? ■ Are there any art objects within reach of the person? ■ Is the door to the lounge room or entry a contrasting colour to adjacent walls or other doors? ■ Is furniture in the room different shapes and sizes? ■ Is the flooring colour and pattern in the lounge room consistent?			

Environmental audit

Unit _____ Date _____ Time of day _____

Issue	Yes	No	Potential actions
7. Entrance and exits from building The main purpose of the entrance and exit door is to enter or leave the building. It is important to determine which door(s) the person should have access to and how to facilitate this access. *Climate* ■ Is seating near egresses a comfortable temperature? ■ Is there an air lock between internal and external doors which allows for adjustment in temperature? *Visual perception* *To reduce accessibility* ■ Is lower lighting used at the door? ■ Is the door similar to other internal doors? ■ Is the door the same colour and finish as the surrounding walls? *To increase accessibility* ■ Is the colour and style of the door contrasted from other doors as well as the walls? ■ Does the door have a glass insert so the person can see out? ■ Is there increased lighting at the entrance and exit doors during the day? ■ Is the door used specifically as an entry or exit door throughout the day? ■ Is there a comfortable seating area for the person to adjust to lighting levels before moving outside? ■ Are entrance and exit doors open during the day in consideration of there being secure areas beyond in which the person can remain safe? *Odour/smell* *To reduce accessibility* ■ Are outside odours prevented from entering the building? *To increase accessibility* ■ Are scented plants or shrubs adjacent to the door or in gardens on the other side of the door?			

Environmental audit (continued)

Unit _____ Date _____ Time of day _____

Issue	Yes	No	Potential actions
Hearing *To reduce accessibility* ■ Do care staff and others avoid standing and talking at the door, which can attract the person there? *To increase accessibility* ■ Do care staff and others stand and talk at the door and describe the outside environment to the person to encourage them to walk outside? **Accessibility** *To reduce accessibility* ■ Is the door pad coded? ■ Is the door exit sign out of visual range of the person? ■ Has the door architrave that sits proud of the wall been removed? ■ Is the colour of the door the same colour as the adjacent walls? *To increase accessibility* ■ Is the flooring between internal and external areas a similar colour and design? ■ Are all trip hazards or obstacles removed? ■ Is there comfortable furniture to encourage the person to sit either just inside or outside? ■ Are the doors automatic?			

Environmental audit

Unit _____ Date _____ Time of day _____

Issue	Yes	No	Potential actions
8. Internal doors – special care unit, utility and service doors The main purpose of these doors is for care staff and others to enter or leave and they are generally off limits to the person with dementia, for safety reasons. *Climate* ■ Not applicable. *Visual* ■ Is the lighting lower at the door and adjacent area? ■ Is the door similar in style to other internal doors? ■ Is the paint on the door the same colour and finish as the adjacent walls? ■ Has the architrave been removed? ■ If there is light coming from a utility or service room into the corridor have the following been done? 　■ remove or cover the glass panel if safe to do so 　■ reduce the lighting level in the utility room 　■ increase lighting along the length of the corridor so the light entering the corridor is not isolated 　■ install a sensor light in the room so light activates upon approach and entry rather than being constant 　■ turn off the light when not in the room *Odour/smell* ■ Are odours masked or prevented from entering the surrounding area? *Hearing* ■ Are care staff and others not standing at the door which may attract the person? *Accessibility* ■ Is the door pad coded? ■ Is the door sign out of visual range for the person? ■ Has the door architrave been removed? ■ Is the door paint the same colour and finish as the adjacent walls? ■ Is the flooring between the two areas contrasted? ■ Is all furniture or seating near the door removed?			

Environmental audit

Unit _____ Date _____ Time of day _____

Issue	Yes	No	Potential actions
9. Corridors can help orientate the person *Climate* ■ Is the temperature regularly checked to ensure it is comfortable for the person? *Visual perception* ■ Is the lighting of even distribution along the corridor? ■ Are doors along the corridor, which are relevant to the person, painted a contrasting colour? *Odour/smell* ■ Are utility and service doors along the corridor closed at all times to prevent odours entering the corridor and attracting the person? *Hearing* ■ Do care staff and others discuss art objects and/or prints on the walls to increase the enjoyment of their environment? *Accessibility* ■ Does the colour of the corridor walls contrast with the flooring colour? ■ Is the floor consistent in colour and pattern? ■ Are any black lines or obvious joins on the floor removed? ■ Are there seats along the corridor, to provide rest? ■ Are there items of interest along the corridor walls, e.g. prints of art objects that the person can see? ■ Along the corridor is the lighting adequate for the person to see individual prints or pictures clearly? ■ Are different style door handles and door colours used for different rooms?			

Environmental audit

Unit _____ Date _____ Time of day _____

Issue	Yes	No	Potential actions
10. Outdoor areas Outdoor areas have a number of purposes including, walking/mobilising, sitting, recreational and social activities. *Climate* ■ Are there covered and exposed walkways for year round access? ■ Is there seating in exposed and covered areas for year round access? ■ Is there shelter from wind, drafts and rain? *Visual perception* ■ Are colour-scapes in the garden created by selecting and grouping colourful plants and flowers? *Odour/smell* ■ In the garden are there aromatic plants or shrubs? *Hearing* ■ Are there waterscapes that can attract and occupy the person, e.g. fountain, waterfall, ponds? ■ Is there an aviary to enhance the enjoyment of the environment? *Accessibility* ■ Are the outdoor paths unbroken, e.g. concrete with continuous colour? ■ Are there rest points positioned so a place is in sight at all times when walking on the path(s)? ■ Do paths end at a building entrance? ■ Are the fences obscured with shrubs to reduce the sensation of being fenced in? ■ Are the garden beds raised for access? ■ Is there a vegetable garden for purposeful activity? ■ Is the vegetation non-poisonous? ■ Are there items of interest, such as a bus stop, a garden shed and/or an outside work bench? ■ Is there a playground for the person to passively/actively interact with children?			

Environmental audit

Unit _____ Date _____ Time of day _____

Issue	Yes	No	Potential actions
11. Environment and confinement It is important that the environment maximises personal freedom of movement and expression for the person with dementia. ■ Does the environment promote a positive experience for the person? ■ Does the environment give them a sense of comfort and safety? ■ Is the environment meaningful to the person? ■ Is their independence maximised? ■ Is there a secure outside area where the person can come and go as they please? ■ Visual sites like a garden, garden furniture and sculpture, such as water fountains, can increase the enjoyment and interest of being outside. ■ Is there sufficient space to walk around with a walking frame or wheelchair? ■ Are there rest spots along frequently travelled routes? ■ Can the person move easily and freely between unrestricted areas? ■ How often is the person encouraged to do activities outside their own room? ■ Are supervised outings during the week organised so that the person, if able to, can go? ■ Is social interaction between the person and their friends and family members encouraged and supported?			

12. Action Plan

Unit _____ Date _____ Time of day _____

Issue	Actions taken	Goal	Outcome (state timeframe & person responsible)

Appendix 3

Questions and answers

- Module 1: Introduction
- Module 2: The Person
- Module 3: The Care Staff
- Module 4: The Environment
- Module 5: The Interaction

Module 1: Introduction

Question 1: purpose of the book
What **four variables** are the main focuses of RTC?

Answer: (1) the person   (2) the care staff
                   (3) the environment   (4) the interaction

Question 2: dementia
What is dementia?

Answer: It is **not a disease**, but a condition of progressive chronic (persistent/long-term) brain failure.

Question 3: dementia
What are the **two main forms** of dementia?

Answer: (1) Alzheimer's type dementia   (2) vascular

Question 4: dementia
What is the **major difference** between the two main forms?

Answer: Alzheimer's type dementia affects the whole brain, while vascular may affect only one area.

Question 5: dementia
What **abilities** of the person does dementia impair?

Answer: (1) thinking   (2) social and occupational performance
                   (3) problem solving   (4) mood and judgement

Question 6: dementia
Another difference between them is their **progression**.
Describe this from the graphical representation shown (see p. xxi).

Answer: Alzheimer's type dementia is three-stage: slow-rapid-slow.
Vascular dementia is step-like, i.e. there is a stable time between each stage of deterioration.

Question 7: admission to residential care
Admission to care homes is usually **not** due to the need for physical care.
What are the **main** reasons?

Answer: Behavioural difficulties and social disruptiveness.

Question 8: behavioural and psychological symptoms
There are two main forms of **delusions**.
What are they?

Answer: (1) paranoid   (2) persecutory

Question 9: resistance to care
Define RTC.

Answer: RTC is any behaviour (from a person with dementia) that interferes with or prohibits care provision

Question 10: resistance to care
Give one example of each **type of RTC**, from the RTC scale.
(Note that there is an increasing risk of injury to care staff as the ratings increase.)

Answer: RTC 1: (refer to section) RTC 2: (refer to section)
RTC 3: (refer to section) RTC 4: (refer to section)

Question 11: resistance to care
Which activities do you have to be **most careful** with in terms of exposure to RTC?

Answer: (1) repositioning in bed (2) assisting with eating/meals
(3) showering/bathing (4) changing/dressing
(5) toileting

Question 12: duration of behaviour
How long, on average, are most RTC incidents?

Answer: 1–5 minutes (60%).

Question 13: incident and injury triangle
Explain the difference between:

■ Minor and significant **incidents**
■ Minor and significant **injuries**

Give your own example of each.

Answer: The difference between a minor and significant **incident** is: a minor incident is where the risk of loss or injury is low, whereas a major incident is where the risk of loss is high.

The difference between a minor injury and a major injury is: minimal injury/harm compared to major injury/harm from an event.

Question 14: incident and injury triangle
Why is it important to report **minor incidents**?

Answer: It can reduce the chance of significant incidents or injuries to care staff and residents, i.e. the use of SAFER (Spot it, Assess it, Fix it, Explain it, Review it).

Question 15: resistance to care
Explain how you would **reduce the risk of staff injury** due to being grabbed when dressing Molly.

Answer: Check response:
No correct answer at this stage.
Will be asked again in Interaction section where a correct answer is required.

Module 2: The Person

Question 1: movement
Consider how far you can move your joints/limb.
Now consider how far the older person might be able to move theirs.
How do you know **how far** a person's joint can be moved?

Answer: You will start to feel an increasing resistance of the joint and limb.
(That is, you will have to apply more pressure to get it to move any further.)

Question 2: movement
In what instance would there be **no resistance** to movement of a joint, and why is this important to remember?

Answer: Muscle wasting around the joint, such as when a person has had a stroke (the limb will seem floppy).
This is important because you can easily dislocate a joint or cause other serious injury.

Question 3: movement
Movement is measured in degrees.
Draw a **simple diagram** of a person's arm, showing 0°, 45° and 90°.
(Note: 0° is the arm by the person's side, at rest.)

Answer: Refer to the diagram in The Person chapter.

Question 4: movement
Most people think that the strongest pattern of body movement is square, i.e. if you were about to pick up a cup off the table in front of you, you would reach straight ahead.
In fact, it is more comfortable to reach across, towards the centre of the body.
What are the two terms used to describe this **across the body** movement, which is very important to keep in mind for all activities with people in your care?

Answer: functional or diagonal

Question 5: ageing and movement
List the five injuries and/or chronic diseases that occur with the **ageing process**.

Answer: (1) presence of pain (2) depression
(3) decreased muscle strength (4) soft tissue and bone injury
(5) sensory loss

Question 6: posture, balance and trunk rotation
What is the effect that **posture** has on Molly's **visual field**?

Answer: Makes her visual field **shorter and narrower**.

Question 7: neck rotation
Where do you need to **stand** to be **seen** by someone who has limited neck rotation?

Answer: Stand within their field of view. That is, either directly in front, or just diagonal.

Question 8: posture and walking
If the **centre of gravity** for a person changes, what does this affect?

Answer: Their **balance** is affected.

Question 9: posture and walking (with walking frame)
Looking at the picture of Molly with her walking frame (*and knowing that she has a reduced field of vision*), how does this **increase** her risk of injury?

Answer: She can't see hazards medium/long distances ahead of her.
                She also can't see people approaching.

Question 10: posture and walking (approaching from behind)
Why shouldn't we approach someone like Molly from **behind**?

Answer: She can't see you, might not hear you, and could react unexpectedly.

Question 11: shoulder, elbow, wrist and hand range of movement
Referring to the pictures shown on pages 15–17:
If this is the limited range of movement of Molly's right arm, what kinds of **activities of daily living** would this affect (give three answers)?

Answer: (1) washing   (2) dressing
                (3) grooming   *others*: eating, playing games

Question 12: shoulder, elbow, wrist and hand range of movement
When, in care, might you need to get Molly to lift her hands **above her head** in this way?

Answer: *various*: dressing/undressing, grooming head and face, washing hair

Question 13: shoulder, elbow, wrist and hand range of movement
When removing Molly's **top**, if she shows **RTC**, what might be the problem?
What **special care** do you need to take in this situation?

Answer: Molly could experience pain on extending her shoulder past its range of movement.
                Don't apply pressure to the joint – work within its range.

Question 14: hand range of movement
With Molly's swollen joints and reduced range of movement she requires **adapted cutlery**.
What **arm action** is required to use this cutlery?
Why is this a **problem** for her?

Answer: Her shoulder and elbow have reduced range of movement; therefore it will be difficult to bring the spoon or fork directly to her mouth without leaning forward.
                The leaning forward could also be an issue.

Question 15: lower body movements involving the hips, knees and feet
When people are **sitting** they look much the same.
This can be **deceiving** when trying to assess the older person's actual physical abilities.
If there is loss of range of movement and muscle strength, what **activities** might this affect?

Answer: (1) sitting balance   (2) sitting and standing
                (3) putting on lower garments and shoes

Question 18: visual field/spatial perception
When a person is sitting **slouched sideways** in a chair, the brain **adjusts** this view of the world to being **normal**.
Older people with **dementia**, who have had a **stroke**, will **resist** being sat up straight. Why do you think this is?

Answer: Their spatial perception has been skewed left or right.
That is, they think they are being tipped over.

Question 19: reflexes
What is an **innate reflex**?

Answer: An involuntary reflex that we are born with.

Question 20: reflexes
A person is **holding** a safety rail. How would you get them to release their grip, **other than** peeling their fingers back?

Answer: Lightly stroke the back of the hand with a tissue or cotton ball, whilst distracting them with something (a comment, perhaps).

Question 21: reflexes
Describe two reflexes that can be used to elicit an eating **response**?

Answer: (1) a rooting reflex (tickle the cheek)
(2) a sucking reflex (put food on the top lip)

Question 22: reflexes
How would you get someone to uncross their legs **without** physically pulling the legs apart? Where should you **position** yourself for this?

Answer: Tickle their foot.
You should stand at the end of the foot that is **crossed over the top** (this means you are out of the way of a kick).

Module 3: The Care Staff

Question 1: contextual interaction (CI)
What is **contextual interaction**?

Answer: CI is a form of communication that is holistic, person-centred, and dementia specific.

Question 2: contextual interaction (CI)
What are the **three parts** of contextual interaction?

Answer: (1) verbal communication   (2) non-verbal communication
(3) environment: physical/temporal

Question 3: dementia and communication
What can happen to the **awareness** of someone with dementia?

Answer: **Heightened** awareness of **non-verbal** communication and increased **sensitivity** to others' **emotions**.

Question 4: dementia and communication
In dementia care, why is **verbal** communication a relatively **ineffective** form of communication?

Answer: The person with dementia has a **reduced** capacity to **interpret** verbal communication.

Question 5: contextual communication (CC)
What are the **four strategies** in contextual communication?

Answer: (1) visual   (2) auditory/verbal
(3) touch   (4) emotion

Question 6: contextual communication (CC)
Name **two neutral places** to touch a person.

Answer: (1) hand or arm   (2) foot

Question 7: contextual communication (CC)
Why should you use a **person's name first** when addressing them?

Answer: They may not know you are talking to them, even if it might be obvious to you.

Question 8: contextual communication (CC)
What are the **five key** verbal communication **strategies**?

Answer: (1) **Person's name first**, and tell them who you are.
(2) Identify **key words** in the care activity and repeat them.
(3) Identify key **emotive words** in the care activity and repeat these.
(4) Use **non-word sounds** to convey ideas.
(5) Constant use of **appropriate** tone, pitch, volume and rate of speech.

Question 9: contextual communication (CC)
Give two examples of **non-word sounds** you can use to convey ideas.

Answer:　(1) 'mmm' meaning yummy　　(2) 'brrr' meaning cold

Question 10: contextual communication (CC)
What are some examples of **emotive words**?

Answer:　*various*: snug, warm, safe, etc.

Question 11: contextual tasking (CT)
Read the example on Contextual tasking when dressing Molly.
Give your own example of what you would do for **CT** when assisting Molly to eat.

Answer:　Sit in **front** (or diagonally in front).
　　　　　　Show her the plate with the food on it.

Question 12: contextual interaction (CI) – bringing it together
Describe three ways you would **prepare to interact** with a person when getting them **out of bed**.

Answer:　(1) Establish in your mind what needs to be achieved, and the order you will do it.
　　　　　　(2) Prepare emotionally, and set the mood.
　　　　　　(3) Prepare your focus on the interaction, rather than on other concerns.

Question 13: contextual interaction (CI) – bringing it together
To **physically approach** a person to get them out of bed what should you do?

Answer:　(1) Approach from the front – in their visual range.
　　　　　　(2) Physically gain the person's attention prior to talking to them.
　　　　　　(3) Use the person's preferred name first.
　　　　　　(4) Tell the person who you are.
　　　　　　(5) Speak slowly, clearly and with moderate tone.
　　　　　　(6) Present one idea at a time with a logical sequence.

Question 14: contextual interaction (CI) – bringing it together
What is the name of the technique of placing your hands on the person's elbow and wrist?

Answer:　Forearm placement technique.

Question 15: standard positioning
Describe your **position and approach** to a **standing** person.

Answer:　Approach directly or almost directly in front of them, then move to a diagonal or
　　　　　　the side of the person.

Question 16: standard positioning
Describe your **position and approach** to a **sitting** person.

Answer:　Squat and diagonal angle.

Question 17: checking the response during the interaction
Often a care staff member will continue the interaction **unaltered** even though the person is resisting care.
What two things should you be **sensitive** to in this situation?

Answer: The person's **emotion** and their **response** to the interaction.

Question 18: CI: assisting to eat
Read the example of CI assisting to eat and describe one thing the care staff member did in each area of CI.

Answer: Example: used key words, smiled, showed Molly the food.

Question 19: CI: language
Refer to the Language diagram, and draw your own diagram using the **specific descriptors** for dressing a person.

Answer: shirt, trousers, pants, sock, shoe, jumper, cardigan.

Question 20: reporting
Read the section on reporting.
Write a record of a resistive episode during repositioning in bed using all seven reporting criteria.

Answer:
(1) date and time
(2) care activity and location
(3) describe the person's behaviour using the specific descriptors
(4) duration of behaviours in minutes
(5) weight the severity and intensity of the behaviour
(6) describe intervention used and effectiveness
(7) initial and designation

Question 21: lifestyle activities
Describe six activities that you could use as part of a normal care routine.

Answer: any six from the list.

Module 4: The Environment

Question 1: creating a sensitive environment for the person with dementia
What is the difference between the **physical** and **temporal** environment?

Answer: **Physical**: built/furnished surroundings
Temporal: interaction with the surroundings (routines, care staff, visitors, family, etc.)

Question 2: creating a sensitive environment for the person with dementia
List three things about a person with dementia that you need to be **sensitive** to when considering their **environment**.

Answer: (1) memory
(2) cognition – problem-solving skills
(3) language
   others: activities of daily living, coordination skills and physical ability, mood and behaviour

Question 3: environmental audit
(This activity can be done individually or with a partner.)
You need to conduct an **environmental audit** for two people with dementia, who are quite different in their presentation. That is:

■ Select one older person who is bed/chair bound and in the third stage of dementia
■ Select another who is mobile and in the first or second stage of dementia

Read the introduction of the Environment so that you are aware of how it affects the person, and then complete an audit for each of the selected people.

Note that when auditing, you should put yourself physically where the older person would sit or stand to enable you to view their world.

Use Molly as an example. She is 153cm, stooped forward, and with limited range of movement.
Assume her position in the bedroom to see how she would view her environment, e.g. sit on her chair and note what she would see/hear/smell.
The sit in the dining room in her regular place and note what she would see/hear/smell.

Question 4: reflection on the environmental audit
(To be done individually.)
Write a **short reflection** discussing what you found in the audit of your two people with dementia. The types of things you might include are:

■ What went through your mind as you were completing the audit?
■ What were the **good things** about the environment?
■ Were there any **issues** with odours/sound/lighting etc?
■ Is it possible to **change** any of these to improve things for the older person with dementia?

Ask your supervisor/educator to read your reflection, and discuss your thoughts and findings with them.

Module 5: The Interaction

Question 1: grabbing safety rail
What are three things that Rachael does to **release** Angela's **grip** on the rail?

Answer: (1) She gently **strokes** the back of the hand and arm.
                (2) She inserts a **soft object** into Angela's hand.
                (3) She uses **key words** to describe what she's doing.

Question 2: cocooning
Describe the possible **triggers** for the person with dementia grabbing something when being sat up in bed.

Answer: (1) lack of **security**
                (2) the sensation of **falling**
                (3) to **balance** themselves
                (4) fright or **anxiety**
                (5) **misunderstanding** of the care interaction

Question 3: cocooning
The interaction: briefly describe the process of **cocooning**.
What is the **reason** for doing it?

Answer: **Wrap** the **top half** of a person in bed linen.
                The arms and hands are wrapped up so that they **can't grab**.

Question 4: mechanical hoist
The interaction: look at the two photos of the visual field for a person in a hoist.
What **approach** should Rachael make with the hoist? Should she bring the hoist directly face front into Angela, or from the side or diagonal?

Answer: From the side or diagonal.

Question 5: stand transfer
How can a care staff member **focus** Molly to put one hand on the arm of the chair, and the other on the walking frame, to stabilise herself?

Answer: Using CI: **holding her hands** in place, using **key words**.

Question 6: correcting sitting posture
The interaction: describe the **techniques** that Angela has used to assist Molly in sitting in an upright position.

Answer: **Repositions** Molly's bottom and feet to the **centre** of the chair.
                She **rubs** Molly's **upper arm** (opposite side to where she is leaning) whilst **telling** Molly to lean towards her.

Question 7: wheelchair mobilising
What **standard position** does Rachael put Molly in to stop her from grabbing?

Answer: The chest hug.

Question 8: applying continence pad – standing
What is the correct technique for applying a pad to a person who is **sitting** and is capable of standing?

Answer: To get them to **stand** upright and **hold** onto a rail.

Question 9: applying continence pad – in bed
Describe in your own words the use of cocooning to change a pad on a person in bed.

Answer: Wrapping the upper body.

Question 10: applying continence pad – in bed
What technique does Rachael use to prevent Angela from grabbing when putting a pad on her in **bed**?

Answer: Cocooning.

Question 11: toileting without rails
Describe some of the triggers for a person **back arching** when being **toileted**.

Answer: *various*:
        (1) sense of **falling**
        (2) **cool** environment
        (3) **misunderstanding** care activity
        (4) nothing to **hold** onto
        (5) being **undressed**/exposed

Question 12: toileting
What **toileting aids** did Rachael use with Angela?

Answer: (1) rails on the seat   (2) a shower chair
        (3) toilet seat raiser

Question 13: toileting using shower chair
When using the shower chair as an aid in toileting, what should be the **placement** of your hands?

Answer: With the **butt** of your hand on the **rails** of the chair, and with the person's hands **on** yours.

Question 14: showering
Describe three things you can do to make showering more **comfortable** for a person with dementia.

Answer: (1) **warm** the bathroom
        (2) face the person **towards you** rather than the wall
        (3) offer the person a face-washer or something to **hold** onto

Question 15: dressing
Why shouldn't you pull an arm directly **up and out** from the body when trying to dress someone?

Answer: Their elbow and shoulder range of movement may be **limited**, and the extra pressure can be very **painful**.

Question 16: dressing
When talking about dressing someone, what is **threading**?

Answer: The clothing is placed **inside out** onto your arm, and it is then **threaded back** onto the person's arm or leg.

Question 17: dressing
When putting the **right sleeve** of a cardigan on a person who chest hugs, **which side** of the person should you stand?

Answer: On the **left** (diagonal).

Question 18: putting shoes on
In relation to Molly, where is Angela **positioned** so that she can't be kicked or grabbed during the process of putting on and taking off shoes?

Answer: **Diagonal** front, i.e. side front opposite leg that is being handled.

Question 19: putting shoes on
How **high** should you raise a person's leg when putting on/taking off a shoe?

Answer: **Within** the person's range of movement.

Question 20: punching, face slap, squat kick and hitting with stick
What are the **two standard positions** that Rachael should use with Molly in these four situations?

Answer: (1) The **forearm placement technique** (elbow and wrist).
             (2) **Diagonal** approach (from the side front).

Question 21: throwing
What should you do if a person is about to **throw** something at you?

Answer: **Don't step forward** to take it off them, step away (so that you don't appear larger and more threatening).

Glossary

Term	Explanation
ADL	Activity of daily living, e.g. showering, dressing, eating.
Agitation	Uninvoked state of negative excitement that is observable to the onlooker, e.g. restlessness.
Alzheimer's type dementia	Most common form of dementia, characterised by a gradual decline in all aspects of function. The progress of the disease is similar to a long slippery slope or slippery dip, characterised by three stages, beginning with a gradual onset, followed by a more rapid deterioration, then a slower rate of deterioration in the final phase prior to death.
Anticholinergic toxicity	The adverse effect of certain drugs, including mild mood elevation, delirium, seizures, extreme agitation, hallucination, severe hypotension, tachycardia.
Antipsychotics	A broad range of drugs that affect the thought and motor response of the person to reduce negative effects of mental illnesses, such as hallucinations and agitation. The older typical group of antipsychotics has more severe side effects than the newer atypical group which also has greater efficacy.
Anxiety	Sensation or emotional state of apprehension associated with the fear of danger from a non-specific or unknown source.
Apraxia	Inability to use objects properly due to motor and/or sensory loss.
ATD	Alzheimer's type dementia, see above.
Benzodiazepines	A group of drugs that can sedate, reduce anxiety and induce sleep. The sedative effect is to reduce daytime activity and lower excitability. The hypnotic drug induces sleep.
Cerebral	Pertaining to the brain.
Chest hugging	Arms folded across the chest.

Cortex	Outer layer of the human brain.
Delusion	Fixed false beliefs that are maintained even when others explain that the belief is false.
Depression	Presenting symptoms of depression frequently relate to inner feelings, such as anxiety, flat mood, disinterest, helplessness, hopelessness and worthlessness and vegetative symptoms.
Extrapyramidal side effects	Side effects of antipsychotic drugs, such as physical (motor) and psychological restlessness, tremor, subjective feeling of muscular rigidity and dystonias, such as protrusion or twisting of the tongue, forced opening of the jaw, spasm in the neck, twisting of the body.
Frontotemporal dementia	Personality changes and the atrophy of the frontal and temporal lobes of the brain. Characterised by social and behavioural disinhibition, loss of social connectiveness to others, and high levels of disinterest and lack of energy.
Hallucination	Sensory perceptions where there is no corresponding stimulation of the sensory organ, e.g. hearing voices when no one is speaking.
Innate reflex	Natural reflexes that humans are born with and generally disappear by 18 months of age.
Insomnia	Prolonged sleep disturbance.
Labile mood	Emotional instability, alternating states of mood, e.g. happy then sad over a short period of time.
Lewy bodies, dementia	Dementia with Lewy bodies is characterised by a fluctuating course of cognitive impairment with visual or auditory hallucinations, extrapyramidal symptoms with a slow progression to severe dementia.
Outflow obstruction	Obstruction of the urinary passage, usually the neck of the bladder, which obstructs or interferes with passing of urine.
Postural hypotension	Low blood pressure that occurs upon a change in the position of the body, e.g. from sitting to standing.
Psychomotor impairment	A loss or reduction in the thought processes associated with physical action.
Psychotropic	See antipsychotic.
Resistance to care RTC	Any behavioural symptom exhibited by a person with dementia, occurring upon commencement or during care that interferes with or prohibits care provision.

Spatial perception	Spatial perception is comprised of two parts: (1) The person's understanding of space in relation to them, such as the position of objects, their distance, near/far, height/width and angles, the depth of the space, colours and contrast. (2) The interpretation of the nature of space. Where am I? Is it safe? Have I been here before?
Tardive dyskinesia	A delayed effect of antipsychotic drugs characterised by abnormal, involuntary, irregular worm-like movements of muscles of head, limbs and trunk.
Temporal environment	The temporal environment refers to the impact of people, such as those working, living, or visiting, on the person with dementia. An example is cleaning routines and their associated noise.
Threading	The technique of a care staff member turning a garment inside out by rolling it back onto their own arm, then holding the older person's hand or foot and rolling the garment onto the person's limb.
Urinary output	The amount of urine passed, usually measured over a period of time, e.g. 24 hours.
Urge urinary incontinence	The involuntary and accidental loss of urine where the older person is aware of the sensation and need to urinate but is not able to hold the urine to get to the toilet. This condition is usually accompanied by urgency.
Urgency	A sudden, strong and intense desire to urinate.
Vascular dementia	Dementia associated with blockages in blood supply to part(s) of the brain. These blockages result in irreversible damage to areas of the brain.

Index

D

E

T

U

V

W